An Entry Level Co

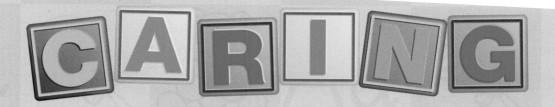

Liam Clarke
Margaret White
Karen Rowell

Published in 2002 by:
Nelson Thornes Ltd
Delta Place
27 Bath Road
CHELTENHAM
GL53 7TH
United Kingdom

02 03 04 05 06/ 10 9 8 7 6 5 4 3 2 1

A catalogue record for this book is available from the British Library

ISBN 07487 6358 9

Illustrations by Alex Machin and Angela Lumley

Cartoons by Shaun Williams and Alex Machin

Page make-up by GreenGate Publishing Services

Printed and bound in Italy by Canale

Contents

Introduction

Both the instinct to care and the need to be cared for are present within each one of us. The question of how to care effectively can be tackled in many complex ways but the instinct and the need are the essence; without these there is no basis. This Entry Level text is a starting point; it explains some of the main points of effective care for those who may just be beginning to think about work in health and social care or for those simply interested in caring.

It is useful as a working text for Entry Level or as a preparation or supplementary text for Foundation Level.

Acknowledgements

Fran Chapman, friend and colleague, for help and advice.

PICTURE CREDITS
pp. 40, 48 © John Birdsall
p.106 © Getty Images/Leland Bobbe
p.109 © Christa Stadtler/Photofusion
Every effort has been made to contact copyright holders, and we apologise if any have been overlooked.

1 Health and Safety

What is covered in this chapter?

- Health and safety in the workplace
- Health and safety in care environments
- Hazards and risk assessment
- Hazards in care environments
- Fire

This chapter will introduce you to some of the health and safety issues that could affect you when you begin work or to live a more independent life. There are a number of reasons why health and safety rules are needed:

- to help prevent injury to people, or damage to their health;
- to tell employers and employees what they must do to ensure a safe workplace;
- to prevent individuals and companies losing money through having to pay compensation or sick pay to injured workers;
- to ensure people can have a workplace where they are safe and free from danger and risk of damage or injury.

HEALTH AND SAFETY IN THE WORKPLACE

Starting your first job, or going for your first work experience, can be exciting and a little daunting, but it can also be dangerous. Every year, the use of work equipment, including machinery, causes accidents, many of

1

which lead to serious injuries and sometimes death. Each year, hundreds of people die at work and many more have to stay off work because of injury. The following table gives some statistics. Most of the accidents listed were slips, trips or falls.

Injuries in residential care homes between 1991 and 1997	
Deaths from injuries	53
Major injuries	4,581
Injuries which resulted in time off work	2,119

Some hazards, such as the effects of working down coalmines or of working with asbestos or drugs, can affect workers' health slowly, over many years.

Because of the risk of injury or damage to people's health at work, the government has passed laws to ensure that employers make the workplace safer. One of the most important laws is the Health and Safety at Work Act 1974.

Rights and responsibilities in the workplace or the community

Health and Safety at Work Act (HASAWA) 1974
The Health and Safety at Work Act is the law that controls health and safety in the workplace. Employers (the person you work for) and employees (you) have responsibilities under this law to protect the health and safety of yourselves and other people.

Responsibilities of the employer
The employer must:
- Make the workplace safe and free of health risks. The employer should ensure, for example, that:
  - furniture is placed so that sharp corners do not present a danger to anyone;
  - there is good ventilation in all rooms, especially bathrooms, toilets and bedrooms;
  - there is a thermometer in rooms where temperature control is important, such as areas where the elderly and the very young are cared for;
  - lighting is adequate.

┌─────────────────────────────┐
│   │
│   LOW FLAMMABILITY TO   │
│   BS 5722   │
│   │
└─────────────────────────────┘

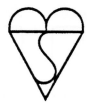

Kite mark – the goods have
been made to the correct
British Standard

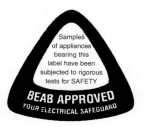

BEAB Mark of Safety – The goods meet government safety
regulations for domestic electrical appliances
(BEAB = British Electrotechnical Approvals Board)

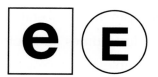

E mark – the goods comply
with European regulations

Labels which show that equipment meets safety standards

- Make sure that the workplace, furniture and fittings are kept clean. The employer should ensure that:
  - all rubbish and waste food are regularly removed;
  - all spillages are cleaned up immediately;
  - dirty linen is stored appropriately;
  - dressings and medicines are disposed of according to instructions.

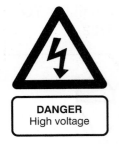
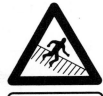
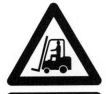
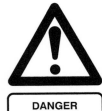

DANGER
High voltage

DANGER
Fragile roof

DANGER
Fork lift
trucks

DANGER
Polluted water

Warning signs should be clearly displayed

- Make sure that any equipment is safe to use and provide details of how to work safely with it. The employer should ensure that:
  - instructions or training are given before an employee uses machinery or equipment that is necessary to do the job (this may be a case of giving the employee manufacturers' instructions or manuals, or it may involve a short training course);
  - employees should never use machinery or equipment unless trained to do so.
- Make sure that any dangerous equipment or substances (e.g. poisons, drugs, cleaning fluids) are moved, stored and used safely. The employer should ensure that:
  - drugs are stored and used in a way as to minimise health risks;
  - employees are informed of any possible harmful effects of using such equipment or substances.
- Keep dust, fumes and noise under control.
- Give employees access to adequate welfare facilities (e.g. rest rooms, canteens, etc.). The employer should ensure that:
  - there are separate marked toilets for each sex and that they are kept clean, in working order and well ventilated;
  - there are wash basins, hot and cold running water, soap, dryers and nail brushes where appropriate;
  - employees have access to clean drinking water;
  - the workplace is kept clean, and waste bins are regularly emptied;
  - food and drink facilities are available.
- Provide any training, instruction and supervision necessary for health and safety.
- Draw up a safety policy and bring it to the attention of all employees.

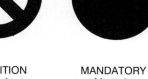  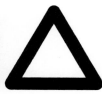

PROHIBITION	MANDATORY	SAFE CONDITION	WARNING
Don't do	Must do	The safe way	Risk of danger
(red circle and red cross bar, for example 'No Smoking')	(blue circle, for example 'Wash your hands')	(green rectangle, for example 'First aid room')	(yellow triangle with black outline, for example 'Risk of electric shock')

Shapes and colours of warning signs depend on their purpose

What is a safety policy?

Employers must tell their staff how they are going to look after their health and safety. This is called a *safety policy*. It should contain the following information:

- who employees should report to if they find anything unsafe;
- how to prevent infection;
- the wearing of protective clothing;
- correct lifting procedures;
- training in the use of equipment.

The safety policy can be in the form of a booklet, or it may be a sign on a notice board. The policy should also be available in a number of languages, if appropriate, to make it accessible to all staff.

Sometimes an employer will put up a poster issued by the Health and Safety Executive called *Health and Safety Law: What you should know*. Look for any posters in the workplace and read what they say.

Important rules

- Learn how to work safely.
- Obey safety rules.
- Ask your supervisor or tutor if you do not understand an instruction or rule.
- Report to your supervisor, manager or tutor anything that seems dangerous, damaged or faulty.

The employer's responsibility towards people who do not smoke

Non-smokers sharing the same work space as smokers cannot avoid inhaling some of the tobacco smoke. This is called *passive smoking*. Smoking is one of the main causes of disease and premature death. Tobacco smoke contains a substance known to cause cancer. Passive smoking can irritate the eyes, throat and lungs of non-smokers and can also cause cancer.

Employers have a duty to protect their employees from these hazards. To do this, they should ensure that:

- non-smoking is regarded as normal in the workplace;
- smokers are segregated from non-smokers.

The European Union has banned smoking in public buildings, such as schools, hospitals and colleges, except in places that are designated as smoking areas. However, the employer does not have to provide such areas.

HEALTH AND SAFETY IN CARE ENVIRONMENTS

The maintenance of a safe environment and the practice of safe procedures in healthcare settings enable the client to feel secure and confident, which is a key aim of good social care. Make sure you know the health and safety rules and obey them.

Rights of the employee

Employees have a right to have clear safety instructions. For example, what should you do if your work clothes were splashed by a chemical you were using to clean a floor? Could poor design of working areas like bathrooms or clients' beds or chairs lead to backache when you clean them?

You should not work long hours; if you do, you may get tired and injure yourself or a client. Remember that people make mistakes when they are tired.

You must be able to work safely, with the right equipment. For example, carers should have hoists for lifting people out of bed or into the bath. You should have the right equipment to do the job safely.

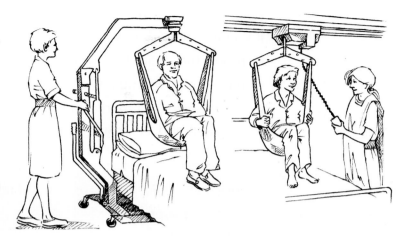

You should have the
right equipment to
do the job safely

Your employer may provide you with protective clothing to wear for certain tasks. For example, when working in a kitchen, you should wear overalls and, if you come into contact with food, you should wear a cap that covers your hair. When handling dirty linen, you should wear overalls and rubber gloves to protect yourself from infection. All such clothing should be clean and washable.

Always use protective equipment as instructed. The employer has a duty to provide, free, any protective clothing or equipment specifically required by health and safety law.

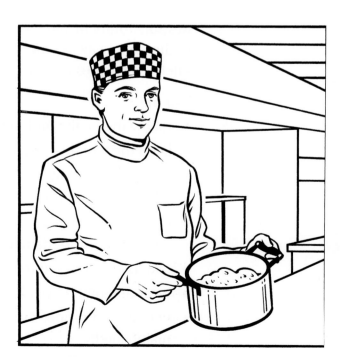

The employer has a duty to
provide protective clothing and
equipment

What should you do if you are injured at work?

If you are injured at work:

- report the accident to your immediate supervisor or tutor;
- record it in writing (usually in an accident book);
- see a doctor – a medical examination should be carried after the accident and the result recorded.

Safe working systems: a checklist

- Do you know who your supervisor is?
- Who do you report accidents and hazards to?
- Do you know the safe way of doing the job?
- Have you been instructed in the use and limitations of any equipment you are using?

- Has anyone assessed whether the equipment you are using is safe for the job?
- If things go wrong, do you know what to do?
- Are you aware of a system for checking that tasks you are asked to do are done safely in the way intended?

Responsibility of the employee

In the same way as employers have a responsibility to ensure health and safety employees also have to keep the workplace as safe as possible.

You must:

- follow the health and safety rules;
- keep the workplace safe, making sure that there are no risks to health;
- report any damage to carpets, flooring, electrical equipment, etc.;
- take part in fire drills;
- test all equipment to make sure it is safe, e.g. make sure that a wheelchair is not damaged before you use it;
- take part in first-aid training in the workplace;
- wear any protective clothing your employer has told you to wear;
- behave in a proper manner so that your safety and that of others is maintained;

- do not do anything you have not been trained to do, e.g. using certain cleaning materials, lifting clients, etc.
- follow the rules or instructions given by your work colleagues

Safe working

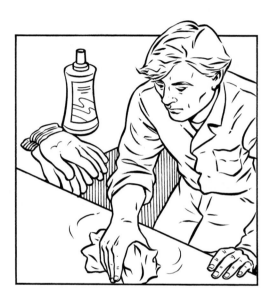

What is he doing wrong?

You have a duty to take reasonable care so as not to:

- injure yourself: for example, a nurse or care assistant who injures his/her back by not using the correct lifting procedures, or who handles certain cleaning materials without cloves or protective clothing, would be breaking the rules.
- injure others: for example, if you injure a client by not using the correct lifting procedure (after you have been trained) or by not using lifting aids.

You have a responsibility to:

- take care of yourself, colleagues, clients, their families and anyone else who may be affected where you are working;
- not tamper with or misuse anything provided by the employer. For example, do not to try to repair electrical equipment, e.g. washing machines, irons, electric kettles or gas fires, even if they are faulty.

As a care worker you should be prepared to:

- dress appropriately for work. Wear any protective clothing you have been given by your employer, such as overalls or rubber gloves. Also remember to wear well-fitting, comfortable shoes;
- always be on the look-out for safety hazards;
- report any hazards or accidents to your supervisor immediately;
- use only safe methods of working.

If you have any questions or worries about safety, talk to your tutor or supervisor in the workplace.

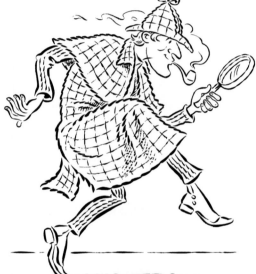

Always be on the look-out for safety hazards

HAZARDS AND RISK ASSESSMENT

How to identify safety hazards in work place (Safety Audit)

Employers have a legal responsibility to identify how much risk is involved in all the things that are done in the workplace. This is called *risk assessment*. The risk assessment helps to identify hazards (see below) before a new piece of equipment or working practice is introduced.

A risk assessment is a careful examination of what could harm employees, visitors or clients in the workplace. The employer examines the situation and decides on what precautions are necessary to prevent harm to people. If this is done properly, no one should fall ill or be injured, nor cause injury to anyone else.

It is important to discover what causes accidents. The main way for an employer to prevent accidents is to first identify a *hazard*.

A hazard is anything that can cause harm, including ill health and injury. This can mean a wide range of things, from something that makes you cough to something that can kill you. Some substances can harm you in several different ways, e.g. you might breathe them in, swallow them or get them on your skin.

The *risk* is the chance, however high or low, that you, a client or visitor may be harmed by the hazard.

Carrying out a risk assessment

The questions an employer might ask when carrying out a risk assessment cover the following areas.

Tidiness
Are all parts of the premises clear of waste and rubbish, particularly:
- storerooms?
- attics and basements?
- boiler rooms and other equipment rooms?
- bottoms of lift shafts?
- staircases and under the stairs?

Smoking
- Are enough ashtrays provided in all the areas where smoking is permitted?
- Are staff advised to use the ashtrays and not to throw cigarettes or matches into wastepaper bins, through gratings or out of windows?

Electricity
- Do all parts of the electrical installation comply with the Institute of Electrical Engineers (IEE) regulations for electrical installations?
- Is the electrical installation inspected and tested at least every five years?
- Are staff trained to report frayed leads and faulty equipment?

Heating appliances
- Are heating appliances fixed rather than portable?

- Do all heating appliances have adequate and secure fireguards?
- Are the staff warned to keep combustible materials away from heaters?

HAZARDS IN CARE ENVIRONMENTS

The employer's duty is to provide a safe and controlled workplace for all staff, clients and visitors. The different things that care organisations do means that each organisation has its own particular requirements in terms of health and safety. For example, nurseries and playgroups have different requirements from a home for elderly people. Each workplace will also have its own particular hazards.

Some common hazards in care environments

- Fire.
- Use of work equipment.
- Use of substances (e.g. bleach and other cleaning materials, medicines).
- Manual handling e.g. of clients.
- Personal protective equipment, e.g. overalls.

What can you do about hazards in care environments?

Large organisations (e.g. factories, colleges, hospitals) will usually have:
- a health and safety officer with the overall responsibility for health and safety policy;
- a system for reporting defects in equipment;
- an accident book for recording accidents.
- If you suspect that equipment is faulty, do not use it. Report your suspicions as soon as possible.

Other general hazards

- Unguarded or unsupervised equipment.
- Slippery or broken walkways.
- Loose or damaged wiring.
- Poor lighting.
- Water or gas leaks.
- Blocked doors and emergency fire exits.

- Poor signing (e.g. to fire exits).
- Unhygienic toilets and slippery surfaces.
- Broken tiles and mirrors.
- Inadequate storage for cleaning materials.
- Poorly maintained lifts and elevators.

Things to do

1 Look at the illustration and write down the number of hazards that you can see.

2 Discuss your list with your class colleagues.

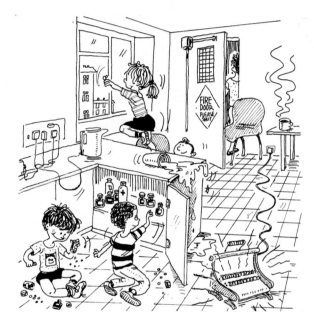

_____

_____

_____

_____

_____

_____

_____

_____

_____

Things to do

1 Note down the hazards shown in the illustration.
2 Draw up a list of potential health and safety hazards that you might find in a playgroup.

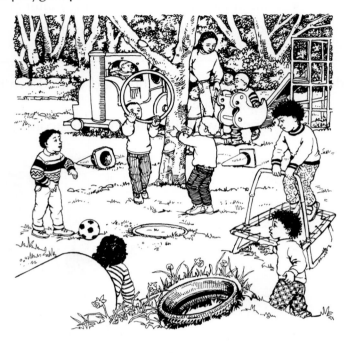

_____

_____

_____

_____

_____

_____

_____

_____

_____

FIRE

The effects of a fire in the workplace can be very serious. Many people are killed each year by fire, and millions of pounds' worth of damage is caused.

What can cause fire?

- Sparks from faulty electrical appliances and open fires.
- Smoking materials such as matches, cigarette ends or pipe ash.
- Cooker hobs.
- Heating appliances such as fires and gas heaters.

What should you do if you discover a fire?

You should notify a senior member of staff, who should:

- ensure that the fire service has been called;
- go to the scene of the fire and supervise the fire fighting until the fire service arrives;
- clear everyone, except those actually engaged in the fire fighting, from the immediate vicinity of the fire;
- order the evacuation of the building as soon as it becomes apparent that fire or smoke is spreading (before the fire is out of control);
- take a roll call of all staff and residents or clients when the premises have been evacuated (a list of absentees from the building should be available);
- ensure that no one uses lifts.

Instructions should be given to caretakers and maintenance staff setting out the action they should take in the event of fire. This should include:

- bringing all lifts to ground level and stopping them;
- shutting down all services not essential to the escape of occupants or likely to be required by the fire brigade;
- leaving lighting on.

You should know:

- the workplace evacuation procedures;
- where the activation points for the fire alarm are;
- where the fire extinguishers are;
- what type of fire extinguishers are sited where;
- how to operate the fire extinguishers.

On discovering fire, break the glass to activate the fire alarm or call someone.

Close all windows and doors.

On hearing the fire alarm, close all doors and follow the evacuation procedure.

LITTLE TOTS NURSERY
FIRE RULES

If you discover a fire:

- Raise the alarm by operating the nearest fire alarm and proceed to the assembly point at the nearest exit (outside the Rest Room Exit).
- Go along the corridor through the Rest Room and out the double-opening patio doors.
- Close the door of your room as you leave and any others you may use.
- Do not shout or run.
- Study this notice carefully so that you will know what to do in an emergency.
- Do not re-enter the building until told to do so by an appropriate person.

A fire action notice

Fire fighting

All workplaces must be inspected regularly by a fire officer to ensure that:

- portable fire extinguishers and/or hose reels are provided in clearly visible and readily accessible places throughout the premises;
- they are maintained at regular intervals;
- staff are familiar with their use;
- fire exits are clear and available for use.

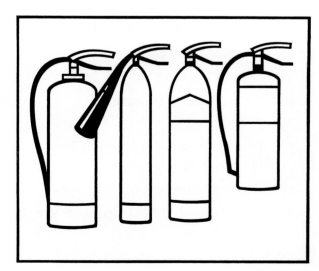

All fire extinguishers should be maintained at regular intervals

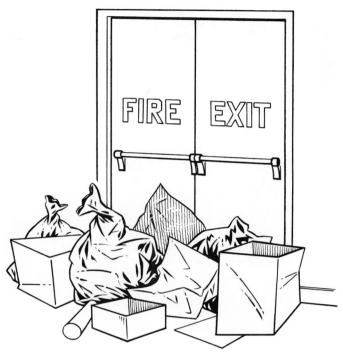

What is wrong in this picture?

Remember that you should only attempt to tackle small fires yourself with an extinguisher. If in doubt, call the fire service.

Things to do	1	Draw a plan of your college, school or workplace. Look for all the different fire extinguishers and water hoses in public places and mark them on the plan.
	2	Make notes of what kinds of fire the extinguishers are for.
	3	Find out what the fire evacuation procedure is in your school, college or workplace. Explain this procedure clearly to your colleagues.

2 Caring for Others

What is covered in this chapter?

- Human needs
- Local care services
- Finding out a person's needs
- Caring for others and understanding their needs
- Skills and qualities of carers

Perhaps you are thinking about working with and helping other people, such as small children, elderly people or people who have disabilities. If you are, you may work in a variety of different environments.

Examples of the type of care settings you could work in are:

- the home of a young child;
- nursery;
- playgroup;
- school;
- special school;
- residential home;
- nursing home;
- day centre;
- hospital.

HUMAN NEEDS

Human needs can range from quite simple requirements for warmth, food and shelter to the more complicated desire to be loved and valued.

Needs can be categorised in the following table:

Type of need	Example
Physical needs	Food, shelter, warmth
Intellectual needs	Learning, education
Emotional needs	Security, love, affection
Social needs	Meeting people, being part of a group, sport

Try to think of other examples of each type of need.

The groups of people you might be looking after all have different care needs.

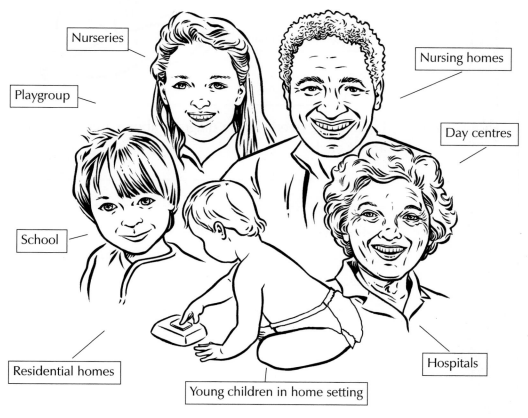

Nurseries

Playgroup

School

Residential homes

Nursing homes

Day centres

Hospitals

Young children in home setting

Working in different care settings will bring you into contact with many different client groups

Babies

Babies are helpless at birth. Parents have to give total care so that a baby can survive, grow and develop skills. The following diagram shows babies' main needs.

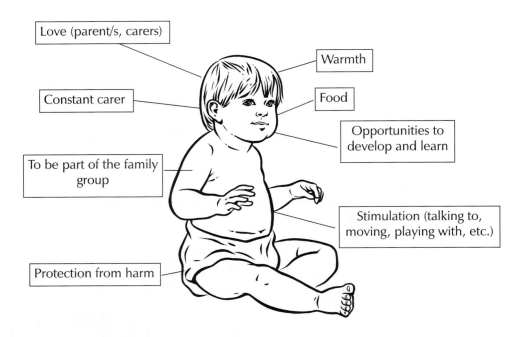

Love (parent/s, carers)

Warmth

Constant carer

Food

Opportunities to develop and learn

To be part of the family group

Stimulation (talking to, moving, playing with, etc.)

Protection from harm

Things to do   Look at the needs in the diagram above and write a few sentences about each.

_____

_____

_____

_____

_____

_____

_____

_____

_____

Older children

Older children have the same needs as the baby in the diagram but the older child will also need to:

- be encouraged to be part of a wider circle of people (to socialise);
- learn through play with adults and other children;

- go to school to promote intellectual and social development.

All children need to feel secure, loved and valued as individuals. Emotional or social problems may occur in later life if these needs are not met.

Adolescents

Adolescence can be quite a difficult time in life for some young people. Perhaps you can understand some of the feelings expressed below. Maybe you have had some of these feelings yourself.

Adolescents have additional needs, for example to gradually take more responsibility for their own lives, but also to be able to return to the family for emotional support.

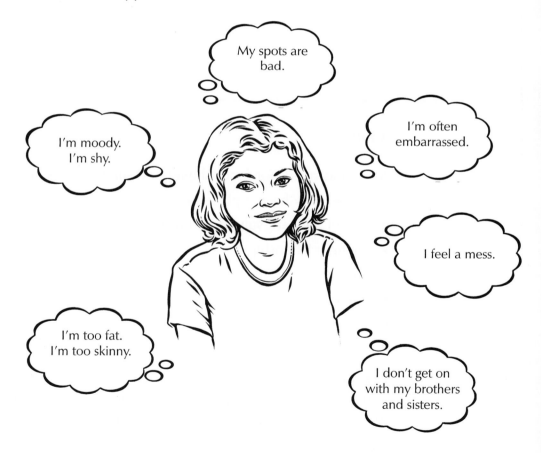

Adolescents especially need to feel:

- included in their peer group;
- understood by their friends and families.

Things to do	1	Write down the two most important social needs of an adolescent.
	2	Think of an important need that you have.

_____

_____

_____

_____

_____

_____

_____

_____

_____

Adults

As well as needs for food, shelter and safety, adults also need:

- to feel they have a place in society;
- to feel they are valued and respected as people;
- loving relationships;
- friends;
- financial security;
- employment;
- a home of their own.

It is also a good thing if adults can feel a sense of achievement and fulfilment, for example gaining qualifications, the feeling of doing a job well, having accommodation and providing for a family.

Older people

As people grow older, they may begin to experience feelings such as those expressed in the diagram.

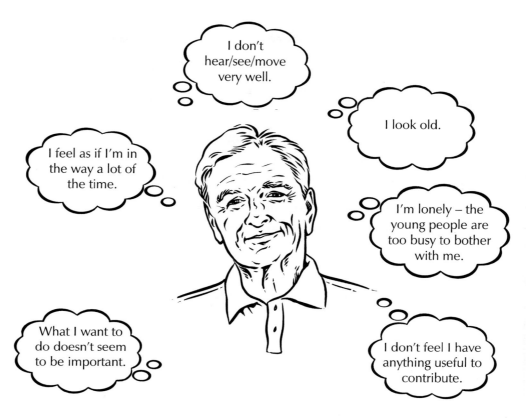

It may be quite upsetting that these thoughts could be going through elderly people's minds.

Elderly people have the same needs as younger people; in fact, their needs are often made greater by changes in their mental and physical state.

Older people have specific needs relating to:

- housing/shelter;
- warmth;
- social relationships;
- physical activities.

However, these may be needed in differing quantities (e.g. warmth) or in different ways (e.g. physical activity) from other groups.

| Things to do | 1 | Arrange to interview an elderly person, and ask them what they think their needs are compared to an adolescent. |
| | 2 | Make a list and compare it with your class colleagues. |

People with physical and mental disabilities

As well as basic needs, people with physical and mental disabilities may also have additional needs relating to their condition. For example, there may be mobility needs or they may need help with speech, vision or hearing.

The basic needs of all age groups are quite similar; however, a person's needs may change due to advancing age, illness, physical or mental disabilities and the effects of social, emotional and financial disadvantage.

As a carer, you will need to appreciate what each individual's needs are and have the knowledge and practical skills to meet these needs.

Things to do	List three additional needs that a person who has difficulties with moving about might have.

LOCAL CARE SERVICES

In your local area there will be a number of caring services available to help meet people's needs. These services will be organised under the following headings:

1 National Health Service (NHS)

2 Local authority social services

3 Voluntary care services

4 Private organisations.

National Health Service (NHS)

The NHS is funded by the government and run by Local Health Care Trusts which plan services at local level. The NHS allocates money to local healthcare trusts (general practitioners, hospitals, the ambulance service, etc.). It allocates this money on the basis of the services that are needed in the local area.

General practitioners (GPs)

GPs are qualified doctors who have undergone special training. Everyone in the UK can register with a GP. People over 16 may select their own GP.

The GP:

- diagnoses (finds out) what is wrong;
- decides on treatment.

Health centres

In a health centre, you will find:

- GPs;
- a practice nurse;
- midwives, who work with pregnant women, assist them giving birth and support them and their babies for a few weeks following the birth;
- health visitors, who take over the support of children from midwives until children are five years old;
- community nurses (formerly district nurses), who work with people requiring health support in their homes. They may be involved in changing dressings on wounds or looking after patients recovering from illness.

Dentists

Dentists offer:

- advice and treatment to prevent damage to teeth and gums;
- treatment to repair damage to teeth including fillings and extractions.

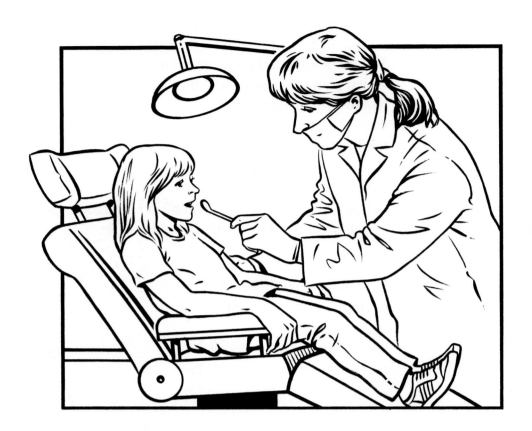

People who work in hospitals

Hospitals provide many forms of care and treatment for patients: this may be, for example, medical, surgical, obstetric or psychiatric.

Among the people who work in hospitals are:

- **nurses**, whose main job is to carry out the care plan that has been developed by the doctors. There are several kinds of nursing, including sick children, mental health and the elderly.

- **physiotherapists**, who help people to improve their mobility, for example after breaking a bone. They also assist with breathing and treatment routines for people with cystic fibrosis to help clear their lungs.

- **occupational therapists** (OTs), who assess people's capabilities after they have had an illness or an accident and work with them so that they can achieve independent living.

- **speech therapists**, who work with people with speech disorders. These range from children with delayed speech development to older people recovering from strokes (damage to a blood vessel in the brain that may lead to some paralysis). Speech therapists can work in clinics or visit people in the community, for example going into schools.

Local authority social services

Social workers can offer a number of services to the client:

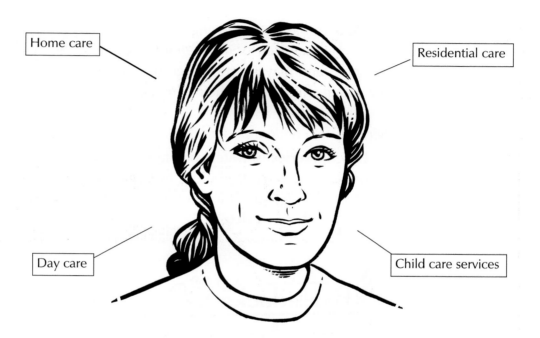

Home care

Residential care

Day care

Child care services

Community-based personal social care
The aim of a lot of social care is to support people living in their own homes. The range of workers who provide this support includes:

- **social workers**, who carry out home visits to support children and families, or older people.
- **home helps** (domiciliary support), intended for people unable to do everything for themselves. This includes support for elderly people, such as housework, shopping and – most important of all – it provides regular company.
- **day-care workers**, who work in centres. Many people who can be supported at home benefit from the opportunity of being with others by regularly attending a day-care centre. This can allow the home-based carer to have some time to himself or herself, or to go to work.

- **childminders** and those who work in nurseries, allowing parents to go out to work.
- **workers in sheltered workshops**, which provide a halfway stage for some people with disabilities. They provide an opportunity to learn and develop skills, whether they are skills of daily living or skills associated with employment. Employment in sheltered workshops both provides an income and builds self-confidence in the people working there.

Services for babies and young children

Early-years services for children include pre-school education such as nurseries and playgroups. Playgroups or crèches provide important support for young children and their parents.

Services for children under eight

- **Day nurseries** (private, voluntary and local authority) look after children under five; they may be run by Social Services or Education Departments. Voluntary groups, private companies and individuals also provide these services

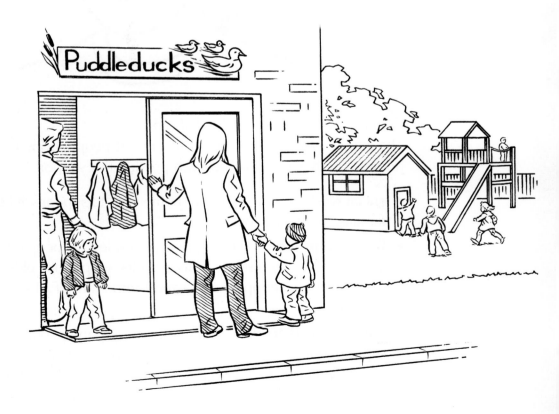

- **Playgroups** provide care for children aged between three and five. Some playgroups may take slightly younger children. Playgroups allow children to learn through playing. Many of the groups are run with the support of parents with one or two paid staff. A few playgroups are run by local authorities, and some look after children with special needs, such as physical disabilities. Most playgroup sessions last for a morning or afternoon.
- **Childminders** have to be registered to be legally able to look after children.

Residential services for elderly people

The largest group of people requiring residential care are the elderly. The reasons for entering residential care vary:

- because they are unable to care for themselves;
- because they wish to live with other people while still maintaining their independence;
- because they are recovering from an illness;
- to give their families or carers a break.

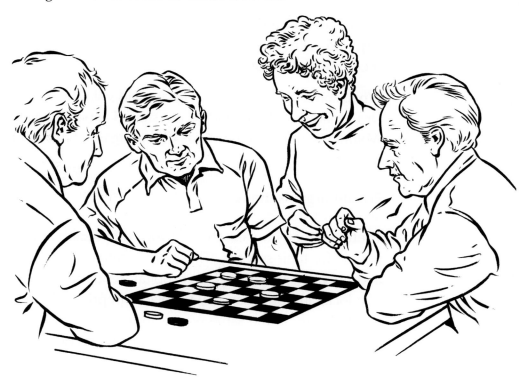

Day centres provide opportunities for socialising as well as allowing carers some free time

Because people's needs vary, residential care also varies. It includes:

- **nursing homes**, which provide care for people needing the support and skills of a nurse;
- **residential homes**, which provide all the necessities for daily living;
- **sheltered accommodation**, where individuals take a lot of responsibility for themselves, and may be almost totally independent, but have the back-up of a warden in case of any problems.

Things to do	Visit a residential home for the elderly and interview a member of staff about the social needs of the residents.

Voluntary care services

Voluntary services are organisations which are not set up by the government. Many are charities, for example Age Concern, the NSPCC, Dr Barnados. Many charities act as fund-raisers to provide for people with specific needs, and the money is then used to buy the equipment or care required. Others, such as Anchor, provide specific residential or sheltered accommodation for people around the country.

While some charities work with unpaid volunteers, organisations such as Dr Barnados and the NSPCC are staffed almost totally by paid staff. 'Voluntary' refers to the status of the organisation, not to that of the workers.

Private organisations

There are many organisations involved in health and social care that charge people for their services. These organisations are part of the private sector and provide services such as hospital, residential and nursing care.
The local authority can pay for places in private homes for those people in need of care, in the same way as individuals can. The government is currently encouraging LHAs to use private services in this way to ease the pressure on the NHS.

FINDING OUT A PERSON'S NEEDS

Whichever group of people you are caring for it is important that you are aware of each person's individual needs. To get an idea of these basic needs, you can look at the typical daily lives of the different groups of people you may find yourself looking after. As the following charts show, they can be very different.

Firstly, look at the beginning of a day in the life of a three-month-old baby. Of course, babies are totally dependent on their carers to carry out all their daily needs, and no two babies have exactly the same needs.

Part of a daily care routine for a three-month-old baby (Full care routine given in Appendix.)

Time	What happens	Need	Response/Outcome
0600	Baby wakes up crying.	Human contact and affection (usually parents).	Talk to baby and give a cuddle.
	Nappy is wet and soiled.	To be clean and comfortable.	Remove soiled nappy, clean baby and put on clean nappy. Talk to baby while this is done.
0615	Baby makes sucking sounds and is crying loudly.	Food.	Breastfeed or bottle feed baby.
0630	Baby is awake and restless.	Social contact and affection.	Cuddle and talk to or play with baby.

Now look at a few hours in the life of an 85-year-old woman. One of Joan's difficulties, resulting from her advanced age, is that she can't even walk as far as the toilet. She never goes out of her house and she cannot see or hear very well. She has difficulty in washing, dressing or cooking for herself. This is part of her typical daily living routine.

Part of a daily care routine for Joan (85) (Full care routine given in Appendix.)

Time	What happens	Need	Response/Outcome
0600	Joan has been lying awake in bed for two hours; she would like to go to the toilet, but finds it difficult on her own. Her carer will not arrive until 7 a.m.	To be helped to walk to the toilet so that she can pass urine.	Joan puts her glasses on and places her hearing aid in her ear without assistance.
0700	Joan wants to pass urine and to have a wash. She would love a cup of tea and a chat to someone.	Assistance with washing. Drink of tea. To talk to someone.	The carer arrives and takes her to the bathroom where she is able to use the toilet and have a good wash. Joan puts her dentures in without help. The carer and Joan have a cup of tea and a chat together.
0720	Joan wants to get dressed and have her breakfast.	Help with dressing. Help with food preparation.	The carer helps Joan to choose the clothes she will wear and assists with dressing. The carer asks Joan what she would like for breakfast and then makes it for her.

You can see from these examples that individual needs can be met in a variety of ways. Support is available from informal and formal carers, as well as from medical and social services. As individuals' needs change, the care plan for them will have to be changed too in order to meet their new needs.

Things to do

1   Write down your own daily routine. This will probably show that you can live pretty independently. Compare how you manage your daily living events with the routines of daily living described above.

2   Arrange to interview an adult who cares for a young baby. Find out from them what the caring routine is early in the morning or last thing at night.

_____

_____

_____

_____

_____

_____

_____

_____

_____

_____

_____

_____

CARING FOR OTHERS AND UNDERSTANDING THEIR NEEDS

Meeting the basic needs of a baby

Although babies do not have many physical needs – just to be kept warm, clean and fed – they are totally dependent upon their carers, so these simple needs take up a huge amount of time. For more information see Chapter 5.

Meeting the basic needs of nursery children (two to five years)

Here are some examples of the sort of tasks you could observe and help with to meet the needs of the children in a nursery setting.

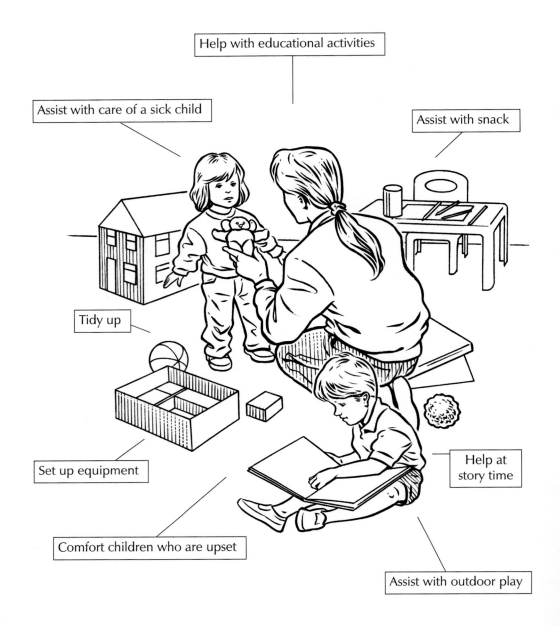

Help with educational activities

Assist with care of a sick child

Assist with snack

Tidy up

Set up equipment

Help at story time

Comfort children who are upset

Assist with outdoor play

Meeting the social/play needs of children – a typical play session
In many nursery settings, a room will be specifically set out so that children can try all the different types of play activities. The room might look something like the top picture overleaf.

The children will need to be supervised and encouraged all the time. Within the session, there will be times when there are one or several group activities such as story time, music, singing and baking.

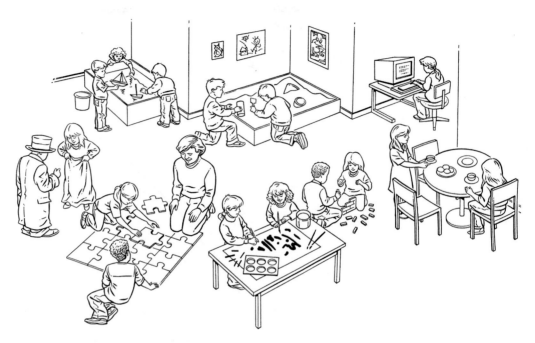

The nursery will be set out so that the children can try all the different activities

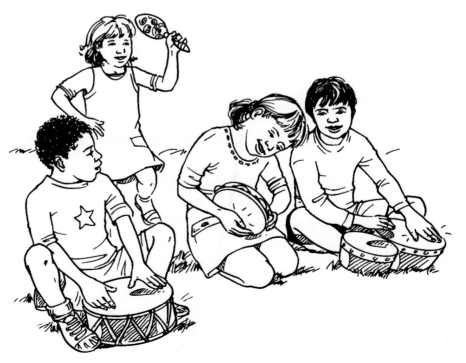

There will be group activities such as music and singing

35

Things to do

1 Think of a cutting-and-sticking activity that would be suitable for a four-year-old child.

2 Explain how you would set up and carry out your activity.

_____

_____

_____

_____

_____

_____

_____

_____

_____

_____

_____

_____

_____

_____

Meeting the basic needs of adolescents

You will recently have experienced this stage of life yourself, so your experiences will help you to understand the needs of this age group. You may also have some knowledge of facilities for young people in your local area, which you can use as a starting point.

Adolescents need to:

- talk to and confide in others;
- be included in activities;
- join youth groups and other organisations;
- help other members of the community.

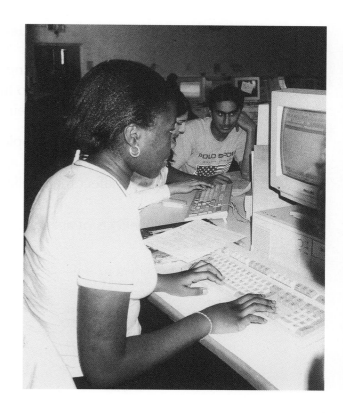

What facilities are there for young people in your area?

You can help adolescents by being a good friend and helping with activities.

Things to do	Write a list of activities and events which you think a 14-year-old may like to be involved in.

Meeting the needs of older people

In general, people are living longer and longer. Retirement age is 65, but many people will go on to live until their late eighties and increasing numbers now live into their nineties and beyond.

Although many older people lead healthy, active lives, remaining independent into late old age, advancing age for some can mean illness, which may affect their ability to carry out the tasks of daily living.

Possible effects of ageing and illness on older people

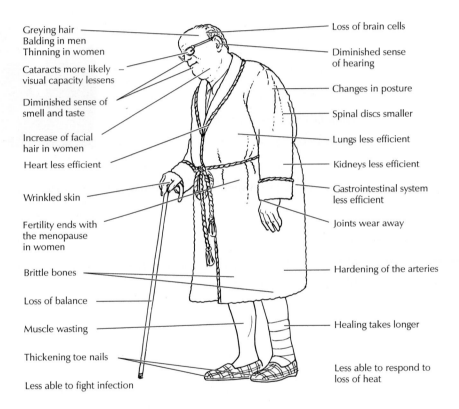

Greying hair
Balding in men
Thinning in women

Cataracts more likely – visual capacity lessens

Diminished sense of smell and taste

Increase of facial hair in women

Heart less efficient

Wrinkled skin

Fertility ends with the menopause in women

Brittle bones

Loss of balance

Muscle wasting

Thickening toe nails

Less able to fight infection

Loss of brain cells

Diminished sense of hearing

Changes in posture

Spinal discs smaller

Lungs less efficient

Kidneys less efficient

Gastrointestinal system less efficient

Joints wear away

Hardening of the arteries

Healing takes longer

Less able to respond to loss of heat

Sometimes, especially as people get very old, more intensive help is required. They may stay at home with help and support or they may need to leave their own homes and enter a specialist care setting, such as a residential home or a nursing home. Those who are very ill may need to be permanently admitted to hospital, while at the other end of the scale, all that may be required is a regular trip to a day centre where social bonds and activities can be encouraged.

Elderly people with special requirements

Some elderly people may need help with:

- preparing and eating food;
- getting in and out of bed and general mobility;
- getting dressed and undressed;
- toileting and continence;
- washing and bathing;
- care of hair, nails and teeth;
- care of the feet.

In your work placement, you may see some care tasks carried out. You will learn by observing, and there may be some opportunities for you to help with basic tasks, such as collecting and washing dishes, giving out drinks, tidying up, dusting, making beds and dealing with laundry while you 'learn the ropes'. Some care tasks, which you could help with under supervision, are:

- serving drinks and meals;
- assisting a client to wash face, hands and clean teeth;
- involving a client in a game or activity.

Never forget:

- to be respectful and supportive;
- to give choice;
- to ensure privacy and dignity;
- to obey safety and hygiene rules;
- to encourage self help.
- the client's rights are the most important thing.

SKILLS AND QUALITIES OF CARERS

To be able to help people, you need to be able to show that you are:

- respectful of the views of others
- pleasant
- friendly
- reliable
- willing
- gentle, kind and caring
- not worried about working unsocial hours

- polite and respectful
- able to maintain confidentiality and be discreet
- understanding and mature.

If you have all or some of these qualities, then perhaps you should consider a career which involves caring for others.

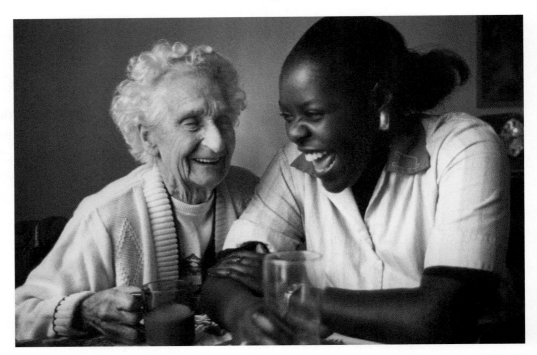

Care values

Our relationships with clients are guided by our personal values and attitudes, what we think of as 'right'. These ideas and attitudes are based on what we were told as children, on our own experiences as we grow older and on what we see and hear around us.

Care values are the standards and qualities carers consider worthwhile when working with people. Attention must be paid to these care values which involve respect for:

- individual rights: the client should be able to refuse to accept the help we offer. For example, we might think the client needs a bath, whereas the client may not want one;
- personal beliefs and preferences, such as culture, religion, food, dress;
- race;

- confidentiality: not telling anything the client tells you to other people without the client's permission;
- the way we communicate with people: for example, the way you address people is important; ask them whether they would like you to call them, Mr, Mrs, etc. or to use their first name. Be aware of the client's abilities, likes, dislikes, etc.

Confidentiality

Confidentiality is a principal common to all care services. Before any information you have gained is shared with other people, you must get the client's permission. You must never tell others anything a client tells you, even in an informal context.

Communication skills needed by carers

To be a good carer, you need to:

- listen and respond to what people say to you;
- use good eye contact and keep smiling;
- be sincere, sympathetic and understanding;
- be kind, gentle and tactful;
- be willing to assist, but always allow the person to do as much as possible for themselves;
- encourage clients to be as independent as possible.

Things to do

1 Take part in a role-play with another person. One person plays a carer; the other person plays a lady who has difficulty in hearing. The carer is asking the old person to select meals for the next day from a menu.
2 Write up the difficulties experienced by each person.

3 Yourself and Others

What is covered in this chapter?

- You and your lifestyle
- Why we need others: why people become friends
- Main life stages: developing good relationships.

YOU AND YOUR LIFESTYLE

There are all sorts of ways in which you can describe yourself. Some statements relate to your character – *I am…* – some to your abilities – *I can…* – and others to your preferences – *I like/enjoy…* Look at some examples of these, all of which are positive statements.

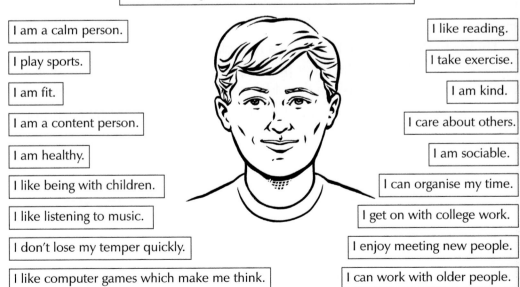

I like going out.

I can see things from someone else's point of view.

I am a calm person.

I play sports.

I am fit.

I am a content person.

I am healthy.

I like being with children.

I like listening to music.

I don't lose my temper quickly.

I like computer games which make me think.

I like reading.

I take exercise.

I am kind.

I care about others.

I am sociable.

I can organise my time.

I get on with college work.

I enjoy meeting new people.

I can work with older people.

I am sensitive, I can understand how someone else might feel.

Things to do

1   Think about your friends, what you like about them, what you have in common with them. What aspects of yourself can you see in your friends? In what ways are you the same or similar? Discuss in pairs.

2   Where do you go with your friends? What sort of places would you go to meet people like yourself? Would you expect to meet friends at any of the following places?

- football training
- fitness clubs
- karate
- judo
- night clubs
- youth clubs
- first-aid classes
- voluntary groups
- Rangers, Scouts, Guides.

3   Write a brief account of your typical day to indicate the sort of person you are. You can mention what you do at the weekend or in the holidays and who you enjoy being with. Make an audio or a video interview if you like. Call your account 'A Day in the Life of …'.

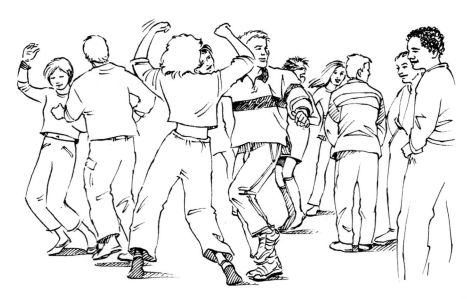

WHY WE NEED OTHERS: WHY PEOPLE BECOME FRIENDS

Humans are social people. Think of the fun you have with your friends or how bored and lonely you feel if you have not been able to meet them for a while. The people whom you feel most comfortable with as friends are probably people who are like you or who like doing the same things as you. People need to surround themselves with friends who will support what they are and what they think.

Things to do	1	In small groups, share a time when you have been glad of a friend.
	2	Make a list of all the good things about friendship. Try to progress the discussion to work out the benefits of other relationships like father/son, brother/sister, husband/wife, teacher/student.

What are relationships?

Relationships can be thought of in two ways. Firstly, there are relationships involving family and close friends, which are very important to you. These relationships are often 'direct', in that you feel you can be yourself. You might do and say things that you would not in an 'outside', or formal, setting. These are *primary* relationships. Ideally, in primary relationships you can be sure of care and unconditional love.

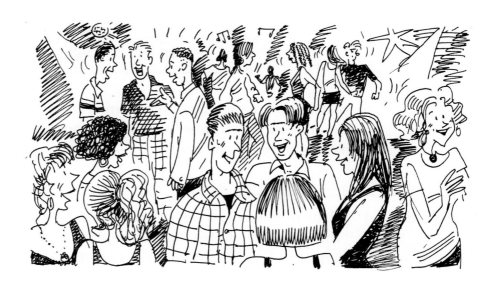

Secondly, there are more formal relationships, such as those between students and tutors (although these may be informal at times) or between doctors and patients. These are *secondary* relationships. In these, there is a set way of speaking and behaving.

Both types of relationships are necessary to manage in society. It would be no good for a supermarket's customer relations if the young man at the check-out decided to pour his heart out to a customer because his girlfriend had finished with him, whilst the queue grew longer and longer. He is in a formal, secondary relationship with customers. On the other hand, if he meets his friends after work, they would think it was funny if he responded to them in the same way as he did to the customers in the store. He is now in an informal, leisure situation with people who know him in a primary way and will expect to listen to his problems.

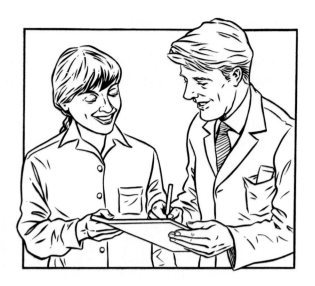

Secondary relationships tend to be formal and associated with a formal relationship, such as that between solicitor and client, employer and employee, secretary and boss.

Things to do   1   Think of some more secondary relationships to add to those above. Then think of possible times when the situation might become less formal and people would act outside their secondary, purpose-specific roles. An example might be a doctor or dentist meeting a patient in an evening class.

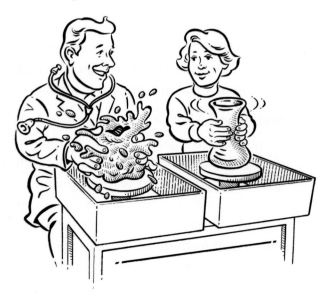

2   Make two lists, one of the primary and one of the secondary relationships you have yourself. Select three people from each list who you like and admire. Write down the reasons for your choice.

_____

_____

_____

_____

_____

_____

_____

_____

_____

_____

_____

_____

Judging people

People respond best to qualities they think of as positive. If you consider kindness to be a good quality, you are more likely to be friendly with people who seem kind. However, in primary relationships, it is very easy to take people for granted and to see family members as the roles they play (or you think they should play). For example, you may see your mother purely in terms of that role, rather than a person with her own needs that have nothing to do with her family. A father may see his teenage daughter as his little girl rather than a young woman in her own right.

With secondary relationships, it is easier to make a judgement based on the role that brings people into contact with each other, although there is no way of knowing what those people are like when they are at home!

What makes good relationships?

One way of creating positive relationships is to treat people as you would like to be treated yourself.

In social care situations, it is particularly important that relationships among staff and between staff and clients are positive. People need to feel good to work at their best, and clients' general health and well-being will benefit from a positive atmosphere.

It is vital, therefore, to know how to communicate with both managers and the other staff. You need to understand their roles and work within those boundaries. You also need to remember the importance of confidentiality and respect for others. When working with those who need care for whatever reason, bear in mind that they may be vulnerable, easily hurt or upset. All actions and communication must be sensitive to this.

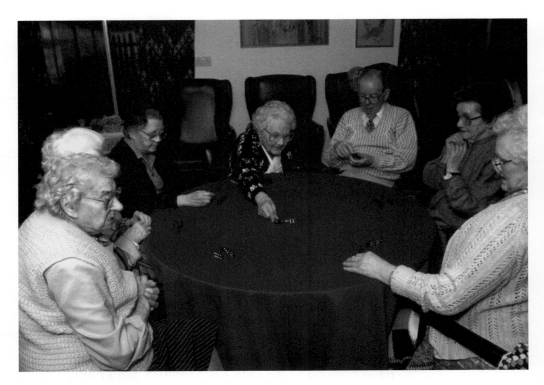

Enjoying company through a game of dominoes (positive relationships assist people's health and well-being)

Things to do

1   Think about the following statements about relationships. Do you agree with the ideas expressed? Are there others you would add?

- Don't knock how I look, where I come from, what I believe in, my family.

- Don't talk about me behind my back.

- Don't ignore me at a club or in the corridor at college. Don't expect me to be telepathic and know what mood you are in.

- Tell me if my boy/girlfriend is cheating on me, but tell me gently.

- Tell me if I'm doing something crazy I'll regret later.

- Don't say you'll meet me to go somewhere and then not turn up because you've had a better invitation or you've changed your mind.

- Don't expect me to agree with you all of the time, or to do what you want me to do all of the time.

- Keep it light; laugh whenever possible.

- Allow me my space, don't push me around and expect me to follow you in everything.

- Secrets are just that: keep them for me and I'll keep them for you.

2   Produce a brief report, written or taped, beginning 'A *good friend* is someone who…' You should also include what a good friend does not do. (You may like to think of someone you know, but change their name for this exercise!) Go on to 'A *good friendship* is one in which…' (Again, you may describe a real relationship or an ideal one.) You should also include factors that make friendships or relationships difficult. Finish the report by telling the reader or listener about *two places* you think it would be good to *go to meet friends you'd like to be with.*

MAIN LIFE STAGES: DEVELOPING GOOD RELATIONSHIPS

These are the main stages in life.

Infancy

Birth to three years: the infant needs care, food, sleep, warmth, protection, attention and instruction. There are fast rates of growth in the body (physically), in the mind (intellectually), in feelings (emotionally) and in terms of relationships (socially).

Childhood

Three to 11 years: although the child has the same needs as the infant, this is a time of continuous growth and development. Many important life skills are acquired at this stage. Education starts in a formal way.

Adolescence

Eleven to 18 years: this stage is sometimes called puberty. There are many physical changes to the body; it is also a time for making major decisions regarding education: whether to stay on at school, go to college, etc. Young people are often expected to do things on their own at this stage and are achieving some independence.

Adulthood

Eighteen (according to the law) to 40 years: this stage often involves a job, marriage and family.

Middle age

Forty to sixty years: family responsibilities increase and then lessen as grown-up children lead increasingly independent lives. There may, however, be increased responsibility for older relatives.

Old age

Sixty years onwards: this stage often involves retirement and increased time for hobbies, leisure and family.

Things to do

1 Think of someone you know at each of the above stages. Write or tape a couple of lines about their lifestyle: the sorts of things they do, say and wear. Make up names for them to keep confidentiality. You could use pictures from magazines to create a 'Life Stages' poster to accompany your work.

2 Write a description of yourself using the following framework. Either work in pairs and tape the responses or work alone and write your answers. Use the words in brackets to help you if necessary.

I consider myself to be … (kind, reliable, pleasant, responsible, perceptive, sensitive, hard working, punctual, smart, neat, fit, interesting, capable). I can say this because … (I give time to the community/voluntary events/organisations, I support other group members, I gain positive reviews from my tutor).

I dislike…(unfairness, violence, discrimination, stupid behaviour, people who put others down, snobbery).

I have strengths in the following areas: …(time management, IT, communication).

It is important to me that I…(continue to play sport, achieve good results in my course, secure a steady job, look OK, meet new friends, keep old friends).

In the future, I would like to…(gain employment, manage my own money, set up home independently).

3 Choose three relationships from the lists you made on page 47. Explain the different ways you behave in these relationships and why that behaviour is appropriate. (You could choose someone from your family, your tutor and your supervisor at your part-time job.)

Ask your tutor to comment in your reference statement about how you interact with others and whether you take the trouble to find out about the likes and dislikes of the people you are working with.

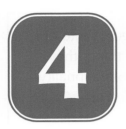

Health Emergencies

What is covered in this chapter?

- Emergency situations
- First aid
- First aid in workplaces and schools

EMERGENCY SITUATIONS

An emergency is an unforeseen event needing prompt action. You can be helpful in emergency situations by having knowledge of basic first aid and how to get help by phoning for emergency services.

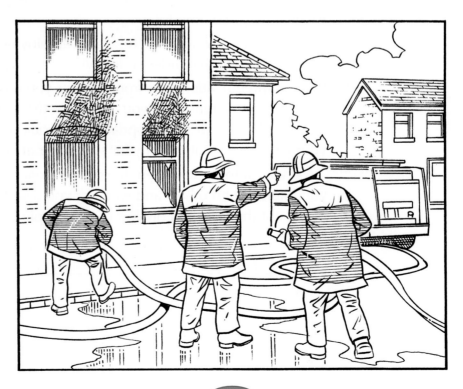

Priorities in an emergency

The key thing in an emergency situation is to help the victims as quickly as possible without making the situation worse or putting anyone else (including yourself!) at risk. You should:

- stay calm;
- assess the situation;
- ensure safety for yourself, the casualty and other helpers;
- identify the condition (if possible);
- get help;
- only move the casualty if there is a risk of further danger.

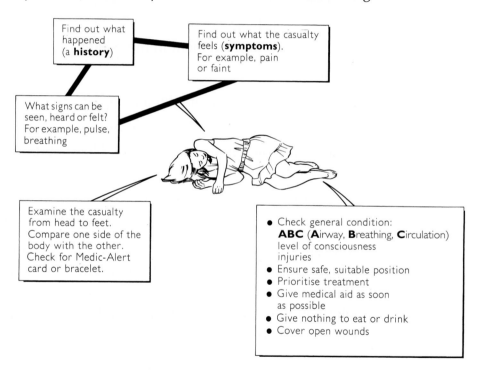

Find out what happened (a **history**)

Find out what the casualty feels (**symptoms**). For example, pain or faint

What signs can be seen, heard or felt? For example, pulse, breathing

Examine the casualty from head to feet. Compare one side of the body with the other. Check for Medic-Alert card or bracelet.

- Check general condition:
  ABC (**A**irway, **B**reathing, **C**irculation)
  level of consciousness
  injuries
- Ensure safe, suitable position
- Prioritise treatment
- Give medical aid as soon as possible
- Give nothing to eat or drink
- Cover open wounds

Getting help

In most cases, getting help will involve calling the emergency services. Keep calm and speak slowly and clearly, bearing the following points in mind:

- If possible, use a land line. If you are cut off, the operator can trace your whereabouts.
- Dial 999 or 112 and state the service required: ambulance, fire or police.

- Give your telephone number.
- State clearly where the casualty is.
- Say exactly what has happened, the number of casualties and the nature of the injuries.

FIRST AID

Despite all efforts to ensure safety, accidents do occur, and you may find you have to deal with injuries. First aid is the immediate help given to a casualty. This may be before an ambulance or qualified help arrives. The aims of first aid are:

- to save life;
- to prevent things getting any worse;
- to produce improvement in the condition.

You should:

- know what to do in life threatening situations;
- know how send for help (see above);
- know the rules about dealing with blood and other body fluids (see page 62);
- know how to record and report accidents;
- keep your first-aid skills and knowledge up to date.

You can learn something about first aid in this chapter, but you will need to practise your first-aid skills. You can do this by taking a first-aid course offered by the Red Cross or St John Ambulance Association. Further information is available on their websites (www.redcross.org.uk and www.sja.org.uk).

Essential first-aid treatment

- Check airway, breathing and circulation (A, B, C).
- Check for unconsciousness.
- Check for severe bleeding.

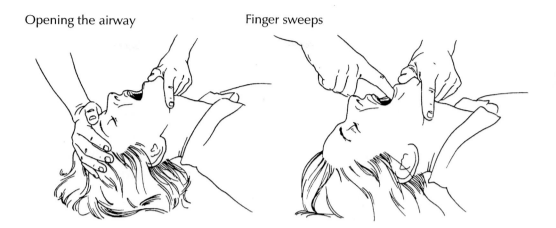

Opening the airway   Finger sweeps

1 Check that the **airway** is clear and keep it open.

2 Check that the casualty is **breathing**. Watch the rise and fall of the chest. Listen for breath.

3 Check for **circulation**, i.e. that the heart is beating. Check for the pulse (heart beat) at the wrist (the radial pulse) and in the neck (the carotid pulse). Use two fingers (not your thumb) and feel for ten seconds to decide whether the pulse is present or not.

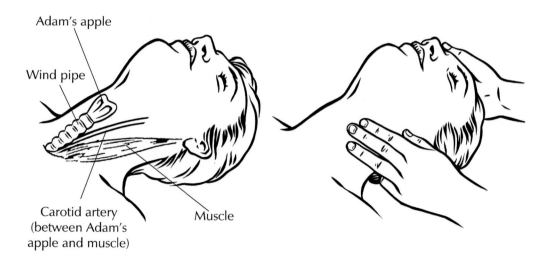

Adam's apple

Wind pipe

Carotid artery
(between Adam's
apple and muscle)   Muscle

4 Check whether the casualty is **conscious**. See if you can make the person respond to you. Touch them, speak to them, call their name. A casualty who is unconscious will not respond to you. A casualty may be partially conscious, possibly moving slightly or moaning. You can assess the level of responsiveness using the following code:

- A = Alert
- V = Responds to voice
- P = Responds to pain
- U = Unconscious (no response)

5 Place the casualty in the **recovery position** (if you suspect a spinal or neck injury, do not move the casualty unless this is unavoidable). To do this turn the casualty onto their side to prevent them choking on saliva or vomit and to prevent the tongue from falling back and blocking the air passages. You should:

- kneel beside the casualty;
- remove glasses and fragile objects from pockets;
- open the airway;
- place the arm nearest to you at right angles to the casualty's body with the elbow bent and the palm uppermost;
- bring the arm furthest away from you across the chest so that the palm rests against the cheek;
- grasp the far thigh of the casualty and pull the knee up, keeping the foot flat against the ground;
- with the casualty's hand still pressed to their cheek, pull the thigh to roll them towards you onto the side;
- tilt the head back to keep the airway open (you may have to adjust the position of the hand under the cheek);
- ensure the hip and knee of the upper leg are bent at right angles;
- monitor the breathing and pulse every ten minutes (write down your observations if possible);
- do not give food or fluids.

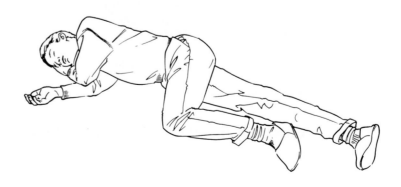

The recovery position

What if the casualty isn't breathing?

Do you know?

A person can live for:

- four weeks without food;
- four days without water;
- only four minutes without oxygen.

If someone stops breathing, you must act quickly. A person who suffers *respiratory arrest* (stops breathing) will very quickly lose consciousness. When breathing stops the patient will suffer *cardiac arrest* (the heart will stop beating) within three to four minutes. If resuscitation is not started immediately brain death will occur. The main way of resuscitating someone who has stopped breathing is with CPR.

What is CPR?

CPR stands for *Cardio-Pulmonary Resuscitation*. First, the airway is cleared, then the rescuer blows air into the casualty's lungs. External heart compressions are applied to keep the blood circulating and carrying oxygen to vital organs.

Look carefully at the flowchart on the next page which shows how to assess a casualty's breathing. Do not attempt to administer CPR unless you have been taught how to do it properly. This is vital, as it is not a technique that can be learned from reading a book. Nor is it enough to have seen it done on TV! You need skilled instruction and opportunities to practise using special models.

Send a helper to call an ambulance at once, or, if you are alone, resuscitate for one minute before calling an ambulance.

IMPORTANT

All these techniques need to be demonstrated by skilled first aiders and practised regularly.

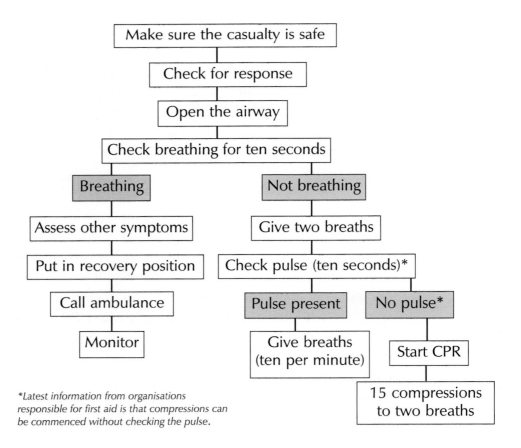

*Latest information from organisations
responsible for first aid is that compressions can
be commenced without checking the pulse.*

Resuscitating children and babies

The techniques used for adults are modified according to the age of the child.

Babies under one year

- Mouth-to-mouth and nose ventilation is used for infants under the age of one year.
- Gentle inflations are given.
- The pulse is felt on the inside of the upper arm.
- Chest compressions are carried out one finger's breadth below the nipple line using two fingers.
- Ratio of compressions to breaths is five to one.

Children aged one to seven years

- One hand is used for chest compressions.
- Ratio of compressions to breaths is five to one.

Choking

Sometimes people – especially children and the elderly – choke on food (or, in the case of young children, other objects they have put in their mouths). Unconsciousness and even death can occur if the air passages are blocked for more than a few minutes. In all cases, you should be ready to resuscitate the casualty if necessary.

The following diagram shows the symptoms of choking.

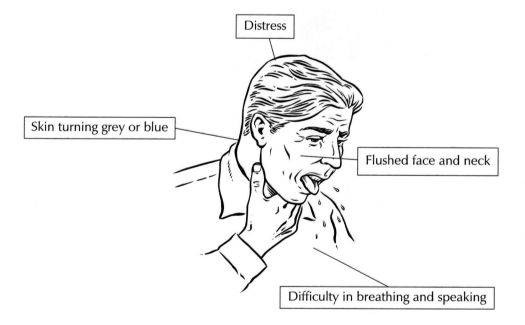

Distress

Skin turning grey or blue

Flushed face and neck

Difficulty in breathing and speaking

Choking in adults
If the casualty is an adult and they are conscious:
- tell them to cough;
- tell them to bend forwards;
- using the flat of your hand, give five firm slaps between the shoulder blades.

If this does not help:
- stand behind the casualty;
- put your arms round the casualty so that one fist is below the ribcage;
- join your hands together and pull sharply inwards and upwards. This is an *abdominal thrust*;

- give up to five abdominal thrusts;
- give alternating back slaps and abdominal thrusts until the obstruction clears.

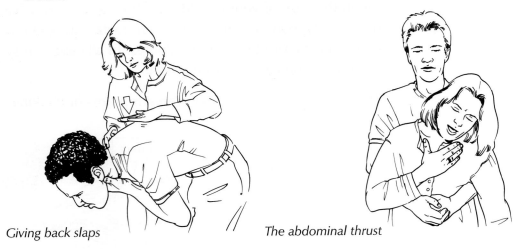

Giving back slaps *The abdominal thrust*

Choking in babies

Signs of choking include:

- difficulty in breathing;
- flushed face and neck;
- strange noises;
- no sounds.

Never feel blindly down the baby's throat, as you may push the obstruction further down; never try abdominal thrusts on a baby. **In all cases, be ready to resuscitate if necessary**.

To relieve a choking baby:

- Position the baby as shown in the diagram opposite and give five back slaps.
- Check the baby's mouth, using one finger to remove any obvious obstruction. Be careful not to touch the baby's throat.
- If there is no improvement send for an ambulance.
- Give five sharp chest thrusts by placing two fingertips on the lower half of the baby's breastbone one finger's breadth below the nipples. Check the mouth again.
- Continue until help arrives, checking regularly to see if the obstruction has cleared.

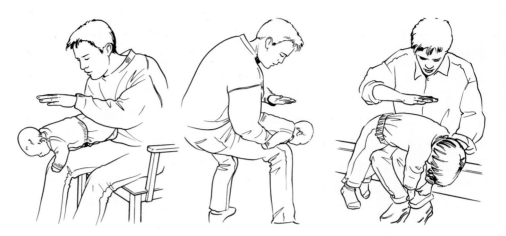

Dealing with a choking baby or child

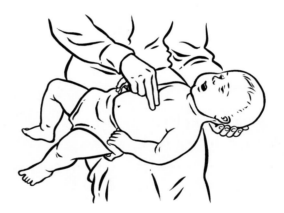

Giving chest thrusts to a baby

Bleeding

It is important to recognise the difference between a small wound that is bleeding a little and a serious wound from which blood flows or spurts out. The word *haemorrhage* is sometimes used to describe heavy bleeding.

Don't panic if you see blood, but you must consider your own safety. Avoid contact with blood and body fluids. Read and remember the following rules:

DEALING WITH BLOOD AND BODY FLUIDS

- Avoid contact with blood and body fluids.
- Wear protective latex gloves when in contact with such matter.
- Wash hands thoroughly in soap and water if you touch blood or body fluids.
- Avoid contact with cuts and abrasions.
- Cover open wounds with waterproof dressings.
- Food handlers should use blue waterproof dressings.

DISINFECTION

- Wear latex gloves and a plastic apron when mopping up.
- Disinfect areas contaminated with blood and body fluids with a bleach solution.
- Dispose of contaminated waste using the appropriate bags and containers.

Do you know?

- The average adult has six litres of blood circulating in his/her body.
- A healthy adult can donate half a litre of blood without any ill effect.

External bleeding

This is usually quite obvious, although it can sometimes be hidden from view by the casualty's clothing. Blood flow can be anything from a slow trickle to a rhythmic spurt.

Types of wounds that can occur:

- cut;
- bruise;
- laceration (torn flesh);
- graze;
- puncture.

Apart from the actual presence of blood, there are other signs and symptoms that show serious bleeding is taking place.

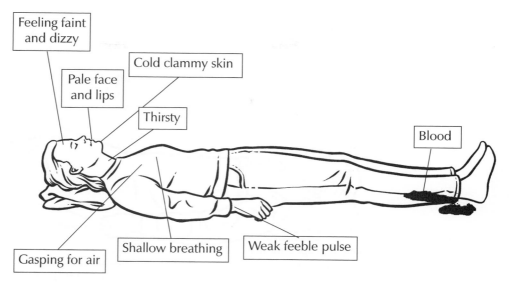

Signs of serious bleeding

What to do if someone is bleeding:

- Get help if there is no sign of the bleeding lessening or if a lot of blood has already been lost.
- If possible, wear disposable gloves.
- Talk to the casualty.
- Apply a dressing.
- Apply pressure to the wound for up to ten minutes.
- Depending upon the site of the bleeding, lay or sit the casualty down.
- If possible, raise the affected part to reduce the flow of blood (see diagram on page 64).
- Leave the original dressing in place, adding more dressings on top if necessary.
- Treat for shock (see figure on the next page).
- Get the casualty to hospital.

Internal bleeding

Sometimes a casualty shows the symptoms of bleeding but no actual blood is visible. This could mean that there is bleeding inside the body. First aiders call this *internal bleeding*.

The figure on the next page shows what to do if you suspect someone has internal bleeding:

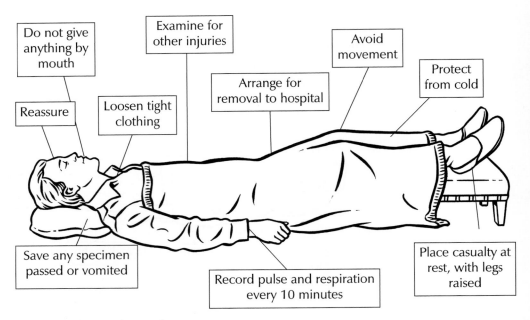

Do not give anything by mouth

Examine for other injuries

Avoid movement

Protect from cold

Reassure

Loosen tight clothing

Arrange for removal to hospital

Save any specimen passed or vomited

Record pulse and respiration every 10 minutes

Place casualty at rest, with legs raised

Internal bleeding: What to do

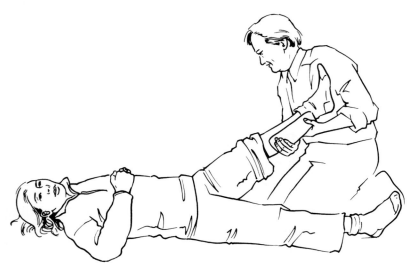

Applying pressure and raising a bleeding leg

Shock

Many people have heard of the word *shock*. In the medical sense, it means a serious state of collapse which may accompany injuries, especially where there is loss of blood or body fluids. A person who has serious burns can lose a great deal of body fluid.

The main causes of shock are:

- bleeding;
- burns;
- diarrhoea and vomiting;
- heart attack;
- severe pain.

A severely shocked casualty will have the following symptoms:

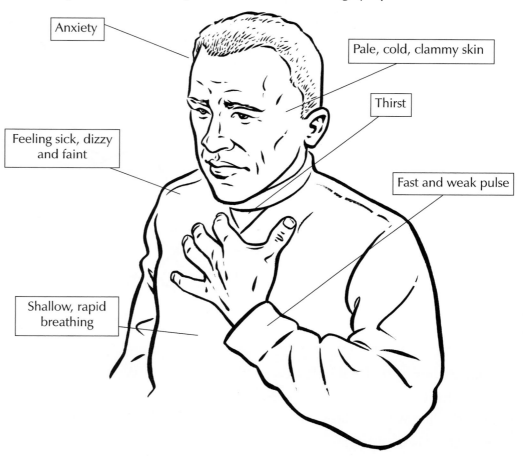

Anxiety

Pale, cold, clammy skin

Thirst

Feeling sick, dizzy and faint

Fast and weak pulse

Shallow, rapid breathing

What to do for a shocked casualty:

- Put the casualty in a suitable position for the injury:
  - minor injuries: sitting down;
  - unconscious casualties: recovery position as described on page 56;
  - chest injuries: sitting up and leaning to injured side;
  - heart conditions: 'W' position (see below) or lying flat;
  - otherwise: lying flat with the feet raised if possible.

- If possible, deal with the cause.
- Loosen any tight clothing, especially round the neck, chest and waist.
- Reassure the casualty.
- Get medical aid.
- Observe the casualty carefully, monitoring pulse and breathing.
- Never move the casualty unnecessarily, give food or drink or allow him/her to smoke.

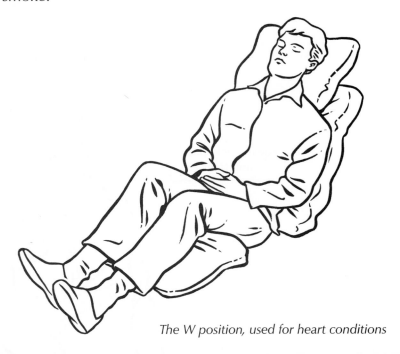

The W position, used for heart conditions

Remember to maintain cleanliness

- Always wash your hands before dealing with wounds.
- Use disposable gloves when dealing with blood and body fluids.
- Wash your hands after first aid procedures.
- Dispose of dressings safely.

Minor wounds

Wounds that don't appear to be too serious can be treated as follows:

- Lightly rinse the wound, with running water if possible.
- Clean the surrounding area with soap and water.

- Always wipe in the direction away from the wound.
- Swabs should only be used once.
- Apply a sterile dressing if necessary.

Get medical attention if:

- there is a foreign body (e.g. glass, steel) in the wound;
- there is a risk of infection (e.g. a dog bite or rusty object);
- the wound is old and is becoming infected.

Infection and tetanus

With any wound, there is a risk of infection. Tetanus bacteria are very dangerous, and casualties are at risk if their tetanus vaccinations are not up to date and if wounds contain soil and dirt. Bites from cats and dogs can also cause infection.

Advise casualties to check their tetanus vaccination status and to see their doctor. Casualty departments may give a vaccination anyway.

Bruises

Another word for a bruise is *haematoma*, which simply means blood collecting within an area of body tissue. Bruises may follow blows or trauma (such as hitting the head against a door); they can bleed, and there may be other injuries, such as sprains and broken bones.

Common causes of bruises are falls, e.g. off play equipment, and sport, e.g. a kick in football, tackle in rugby, being hit with a cricket ball.

What to do about bruises:

- Check for more serious injuries such as broken bones, and seek medical help if necessary.
- Reassure (talk to) the casualty.
- If there is any bleeding, deal with it (see above).
- Apply a cold compress (a clean dressing soaked in cold water).
- Elevate (raise) the injured part if possible.
- Bruising to the eye and blood in the white of the eye should always be referred to a doctor or nurse.

Burns and scalds

There are various causes of burns and scalds:

- A burn is damage caused by dry heat (flames or hot objects).
- A scald is damage caused by wet heat (hot water, steam).
- A chemical burn is damage caused by chemicals.
- Electricity can also cause burns.

Do you know?

- When the body is damaged by burns or scalds, the damage continues even when the casualty has been removed from the source of heat, just as joint of meat will carry on cooking when you remove it from the oven.
- Cooling burns immediately is vital.

As well as damaging the skin, burns and scalds damage the blood vessels below the skin. A colourless fluid called *plasma* (the liquid part of the blood) leaks out. If a large area has been burned, considerable amounts of this fluid will be lost, causing the casualty to suffer shock (see pages 64–66).

Burns and scalds should be treated promptly to prevent shock, avoid infection and relieve pain.

What to do about burns and scalds:

- Cool the burned area with water for ten minutes. Running water is best.
- Take off any tight belts or jewellery (burned skin can swell).
- Cover the burned area with a clean, loose, non-fluffy dressing.
- Comfort and reassure the casualty.
- Treat the casualty for shock (see pages 64–66) if burns are large or deep.
- Seek medical aid for burns larger than 2.5cm in diameter, burns to the face or if you are in any doubt.
- Rinse chemical burns for 20 minutes.
- Do not cover burns to the face; keep cooling until help arrives.
- Do not remove anything which is sticking to the burn.
- Do not apply creams or lotions.
- Do not break blisters.
- Do not use plasters.

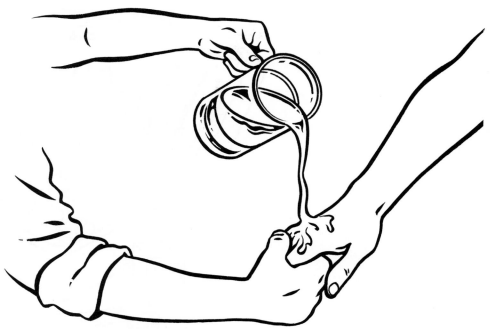

Cooling the burned area with cold water

Sunburn

Remember that sunburn can be a serious form of burning. Avoid it yourself by keeping out of the sun and always protect small children from the sun.

What to do about sunburn:

- Get the casualty out of the sun, either indoors or in the shade.
- Cool the skin with cold water.
- Give drinks of water at frequent intervals.
- If there is blistering, seek medical advice.

FIRST AID IN WORKPLACES AND SCHOOLS

Employers have to be sure that adequate first aid facilities and equipment are available in workplaces. There will usually be a first aid room and first aid boxes will be located in strategic areas.

The actual number of first aiders required depends upon the types of hazard in the particular workplace. A person is appointed to take charge of first aid arrangements. All workers must know how to access the first aid facilities.

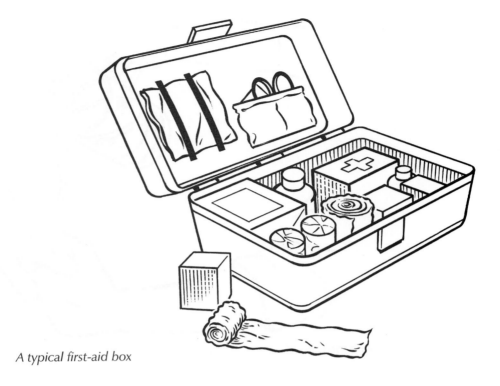

A typical first-aid box

Recording and reporting accidents and injuries in school/college or workplace

What you must do in any first-aid situation:

- Deal with the immediate emergency.
- Contact the emergency services. Get help from other members of staff or the public.
- Report the incident to your supervisor, teacher or tutor.
- Record exactly what happened in the accident book.
- Depending upon what happened, information may also need to be passed to other organisations, e.g. HSE and EMAS.

What does the HSE (Health and Safety Executive) do?

- It investigates and reports on accidents in the workplace.
- It appoints inspectors.

What does EMAS (Employment Medical Advisory Service) do?

- It is part of the Health and Safety Executive.
- It investigates and gives free advice about health and safety at work.

Never forget your own responsibility to ...

- work safely;
- update your knowledge;
- deliver effective first aid;

- gain a Red Cross or St John Ambulance certificate if possible;
- know when further help is required;
- know procedures for reporting and recording accidents.

Things to do

1 Make a list of the details that must be recorded in an accident book in a workplace.

2 Find out more about RIDDOR (Reporting on Injuries, Diseases and Dangerous Occurrences Regulations), HSE and EMAS. Collect leaflets and report back to your colleagues in class.

3 Find out what should be included in first aid boxes in the workplace.

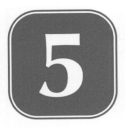

Preparation for Parenthood

What is covered in this chapter?

- Factors to consider before conception
- Preparing for the birth
- The birth
- Adjusting to the new baby
- Caring for the new baby
- Aspects of parenthood

Before deciding to start a family, a couple needs to be quite sure exactly what is involved. This chapter looks at some of the things that should be considered before making the life-changing decision to become a parent.

Although a sexual relationship is the only *necessary* relationship to have a child, a loving, stable *emotional* relationship between the parents is very important. Many people think that it is best if there is a firm commitment between the partners before starting a sexual relationship. Sexual relationships are best established where there is genuine love, affection and respect between the couple.

What sort of qualities do people look for in a possible long-term partner?

SINGLE PARENTS

This chapter assumes that both parents will be involved in looking after the baby. There are, however, many situations where either the mother or father is left to cope alone. In these cases, the difficulties and pressures may be even greater, and more external support may be required.

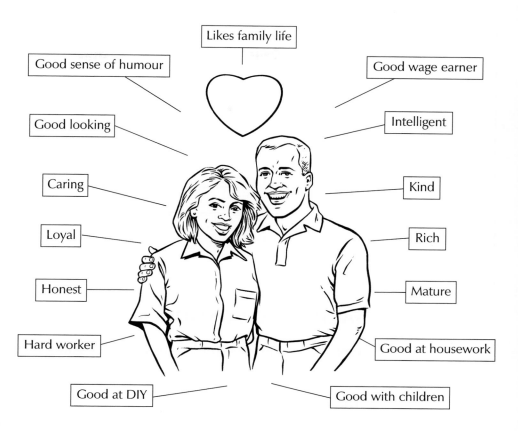

The qualities that people might look for in a long-term partner

Things to do	1	Look at the list above. Which qualities do you think are most important?
	2	Make your own list in order of importance to you. Are there any other qualities you would add? Why?

_____

_____

_____

_____

_____

_____

_____

FACTORS TO CONSIDER BEFORE CONCEPTION

Once a couple have settled into a close, stable relationship together, they might consider having a baby. This is a very big step to take.

The main factors involved are:

- age, level of maturity and emotional stability of the couple;
- employment, money to live on, money to buy equipment;
- having somewhere to live;
- the health and medical history of the couple;
- the lifestyle of both partners;
- knowledge and understanding of childcare practices;
- help and support from family and friends;
- professional support.

Age, level of maturity and emotional stability

Research has shown that when couples have children at a very young age without appropriate support and planning, relationships tend to break down. Young people can be excellent parents, but they do need to be aware of the changes that a baby will bring to their lives. Once the baby has arrived, constant care and attention will be required. If people are in any doubt about what this entails, they should spend 24 hours with someone and their young baby.

In some places, couples can borrow a special doll for a period of time. The doll cries to show when it needs care. Couples are usually quite surprised at the amount of care required.

A couple will both need to be aware of the constant demands the baby will make. Their own social life and freedom to go out when they want will be strictly limited. There will be no more lie-ins: babies wake frequently in the night for feeds and may wake to start the day at six o'clock in the morning. Babies need constant care and companionship and are totally dependent on their parents.

Things to do	Set up an interview with a parent. Prepare a tick chart showing the times of day and ask the parent to record every time the baby cries over a 24-hour period. Discuss the completed record with the parent(s).

Employment and income

One or both partners may work, which may mean making arrangements for childcare. There will be financial implications, as childcare can be expensive. Getting the right care for the baby is vital.

Sometimes neither partner has paid work. In that situation, couples will need advice on which benefits they are entitled to. This is available at local social security offices, which are in the phone book under 'Benefits Agency'. One or both partners may wish to continue their education. The local Citizens Advice Bureau is a good place to visit for information about benefits and is usually less busy than social security offices.

Taking maternity leave
Every woman who is employed during pregnancy is entitled to 14 weeks' maternity leave. When she returns to work, she can go back to the same job. Employers will have detailed information on this.

Having somewhere to live

A baby needs to live in a warm, clean, secure environment. It is best if a couple can have their own home or, if this is not possible, their own accommodation within another home. However, housing is expensive to rent or buy, and not all properties are ideal for children to grow up in, so help and support from the wider family is useful.

Things to do	Make a list of important points to consider when looking for somewhere to live with small children.

Health and medical history

Both prospective parents should be in good general health before attempting to have a baby. Advice on pre-conceptual care is available at doctors' surgeries and clinics. Depending on the family history of both partners, sometimes genetic counselling is offered. This means that the couple will be asked about inherited conditions in their families that might affect the health of their baby.

Lifestyle

The lifestyle of both partners is important, whether before conception, during pregnancy or after the birth. Couples should be aware of any changes they could make for the well-being of their baby and decide if they are prepared to make the changes.

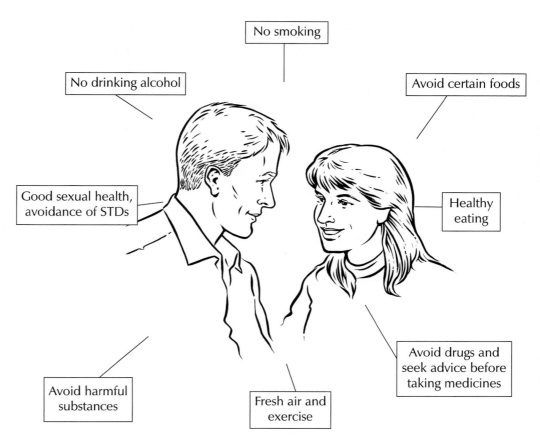

No smoking

No drinking alcohol

Avoid certain foods

Good sexual health, avoidance of STDs

Healthy eating

Avoid harmful substances

Fresh air and exercise

Avoid drugs and seek advice before taking medicines

A healthy lifestyle is important for prospective parents

Knowledge and understanding of childcare practices

Both partners should find out as much as possible about all aspects of childcare. They will need to know about:

- physical care, including feeding, changing, bathing and care routines, and changes as the baby grows older;
- ways of encouraging learning and intellectual development through communicating, interaction and all the stages and types of play;
- giving security, love and affection through all the care routines;
- socialisation, firstly with the main carers through bonding and then with the wider family and friends.

All new mothers will receive the Health Education Authority books *Pregnancy* and *Birth to Five*. These books are packed with information on all aspects of care.

Help and support from family and friends

Couples can get a great deal of assistance from the extended family and close friends. Grandparents can be particularly useful, as they are experienced in caring for children and will probably wish to be involved and be able to give advice. Having good friends is essential, especially friends who have children themselves. Problems can be talked through, and friends' children will be playmates. Many such friendships are forged through antenatal classes and nursery groups.

Professional support

Couples need to be aware of the full range of support available to help them. The key to accessing support is usually the doctor, midwife or health visitor in the early stages. Later on, support is available in selecting types of care, such as childminders, nurseries and school education.

PREPARING FOR THE BIRTH

The mother and baby will receive *antenatal care* before the birth by attending the antenatal clinic at regular intervals for check-ups. The father is also invited to certain classes, such as those which explain about labour and birth.

What happens at the antenatal clinic?

- Meet the midwife and doctor
- Choose type of birth: home or hospital?
- Blood tests
- Urine tests
- Check height and weight
- Medical and family history, including previous pregnancies
- Check blood pressure
- Advice on diet and healthy lifestyle
- Preparation for labour
- Advice on feeding the baby and general care
- Parentcraft classes for both parents

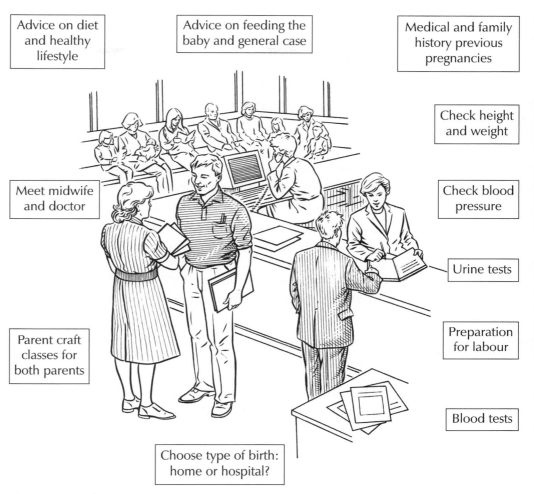

The antenatal clinic

Advice on diet and healthy lifestyle

Advice on feeding the baby and general case

Medical and family history previous pregnancies

Check height and weight

Check blood pressure

Meet midwife and doctor

Urine tests

Parent craft classes for both parents

Preparation for labour

Blood tests

Choose type of birth: home or hospital?

THE BIRTH

Parents will have been asked about the type of birth they would like, e.g. at home or in the hospital, or even a water birth.

Usually the father will be there, but sometimes the mother may choose a different birth partner, such as her own mother or a close friend. The aim is for the birth to be as calm and relaxed as possible. All births will be different, depending on the individual mother, and some stages may take more or less time than indicated here. There may be complications if, for example, it is a multiple birth (twins or more), if the baby is in the breech position, or if the labour is long and those caring for the mother need to intervene for her sake and that of the baby.

Labour

The period in the hours just before the birth is known as *labour*. Labour is triggered by the release of a chemical. There is a show of blood, and the 'waters' surrounding the baby break.

The mother will feel regular contractions ('labour pains').

The **first stage** of labour can last up to 24 hours; contractions become regular, stronger and more frequent towards the end of this stage. At the same time, the cervix (the exit from the uterus, or womb, gradually opens to allow the baby's head to emerge. The midwife and medical team, as well as the birth partner, all support the mother.

The **second stage** of labour starts when the cervix is fully *dilated* (i.e. open, 10cm in diameter). The mother then feels ready to push, and the baby is carefully delivered and, provided there are no problems, given straight to the mother and father to hold and cuddle. This stage generally lasts about an hour.

The **third stage** of the labour is the delivery of the *placenta* (afterbirth). This has been the baby's life support, providing nutrition and removing waste during the pregnancy. It is carefully checked before being disposed of to make sure that it is complete and that none of it has been left behind in the womb, as this can cause bleeding later on.

What happens next?

- The midwife and a specialist doctor will check the baby, if the birth takes place in hospital.
- The main checks include breathing, heartbeat and response to stimuli, as well as weight, length and head circumference.
- A special identity bracelet is attached to the baby in hospitals.
- The baby is washed and dressed.
- The mother is checked, made comfortable and given time to rest.
- Parents are given time to be with the baby.
- The baby may be given a breastfeed.
- The baby is allowed to sleep and recover.
- The baby is introduced to the other family members.

ADJUSTING TO THE NEW BABY

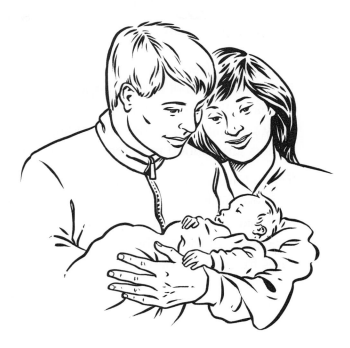

Feelings after the birth

Both parents will want to handle the baby and to feel close. Fathers should always be included. The more both parents can cuddle and hold the baby, the more confident they will feel.

How mothers feel

Mothers usually feel very excited and pleased when the baby arrives and they are able to cope. Some mothers feel tired and a little sore. Three or four days after the birth, about 80% of mothers go through 'baby blues', caused by hormone changes, tiredness and soreness, or even a feeling of anti-climax after all the excitement of the birth. In general, they feel anxious and keep bursting into tears; however, these feelings usually only last a few days. Mothers should have a good cry if they feel like it and get plenty of rest. The rest of the family can give support by helping with the baby. If a mother continues to feel depressed and unable to cope, she should contact her GP or health visitor for advice. Although resuming sexual relations may be the last thing on a mother's mind, parents should seek advice from their GP or the family planning clinic on the spacing of future pregnancies and the most suitable methods of contraception for both parents, providing there are no cultural or religious objections. Contraception will usually be discussed at the mother's first check-up after the birth of the baby.

How fathers feel

The father can feel left out, especially if he was not able to be present at the birth. Fathers need support and encouragement to become involved. They will gain confidence by holding, cuddling and caring for the baby. Fathers are entitled to paternity leave from work after the birth.

If they haven't already done so, both parents will need to discuss their roles and responsibilities towards the new and existing family members. Will they take it in turns to get up at night for the baby? Will the father take over some of the mother's responsibilities around the home while she cares for the new baby?

How brothers and sisters feel

When a new baby arrives, brothers and sisters may feel a little jealous at all the attention the baby is receiving. Older children don't always find new babies very lovable, but they usually find them quite interesting. Often older children may become more demanding when they see how much attention the baby is getting.

Parents can take the following steps to help in this situation:

- Not expect other children to feel as pleased about the baby as they do.
- Along with relatives and friends, try to prepare the children for the arrival of another baby and include them in the care of the baby.
- Ask brothers and sisters to fetch and carry things for the baby.
- Find something special for older children to do at feed times, e.g. read a story or sit close and help.
- Not refuse requests and try to be patient, even if the older child goes back to baby-type behaviour such as wanting a bottle again or bed wetting.
- Try to spend time alone with the older children. Grandparents can be helpful, perhaps caring for the baby while parents are with other children.
- Parents can feel pulled in different directions at this time. Jealousy is usually shown in one way or another sooner or later.

| Things to do | 1 | Ask your relatives what happened in your family when a new baby arrived. |
| | 2 | Discuss ways of dealing with jealousy within your class/group. |

Settling in back at home

Mothers usually find that their immediate family and friends are only too pleased to help with the new baby. Sometimes there can be too much advice given, and people – quite understandably – do tend to describe what they did and what happened to them. This is not always helpful – in fact, it can be quite annoying. Parents will want to find their own ways of doing things; they can listen politely to advice and then decide whether or not they want to take it.

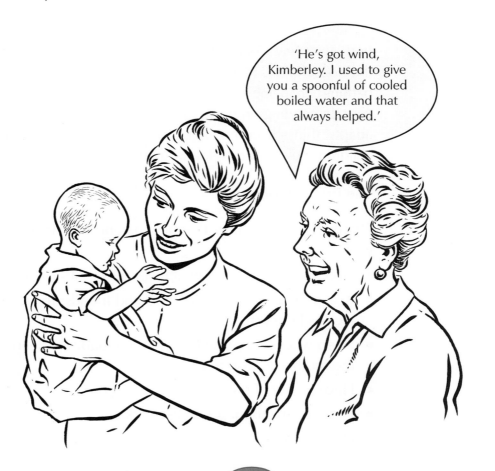

'He's got wind, Kimberley. I used to give you a spoonful of cooled boiled water and that always helped.'

Returning to work

Parents will need to decide who is going to work and who is going to be responsible for childcare. This will depend upon several factors, including:

- preferences as to who will have paid work and who will care for the children;
- which parent's job is best paid;
- whether parents want joint responsibility for the childcare and earning money;
- how many children there are;
- affordability and availability of good childcare;
- help available from family and friends;
- factors concerning cultural traditions in certain communities.

CARING FOR THE NEW BABY

Establishing a routine

In the first few weeks, the baby has to come first, so any existing routine in the household is likely to be disrupted by the new routines of feeding, bathing, changing and playing with the baby. The first few months can be very demanding on new parents, but as the child grows and the family adapts, things become easier. Also, parents gain in confidence as they see children grow and develop in their care.

The first few weeks

There are various things that new parents can do to make the first few weeks easier.

- Don't worry – contact health visitors or GPs for advice when necessary.
- Accept help from grandparents and friends: they can shop and cook as well as help with the baby.
- Sleep whenever possible. When the baby is asleep is a good time for the mother to rest, too.
- Have plenty of nutritious, easily prepared food.
- Don't worry about the housework.
- Avoid having too many visitors; they can be tiring.

After a week or two, babies will start to follow a certain pattern. They will wake for feeds at certain times and be awake and active at other times.

In the early days, some babies may sleep as much as 20 hours out of 24. Others are more wakeful.

| Things to do | 1 | Discuss the daily care routine with a mother of a baby. |
| | 2 | Decide whether you think having a routine of some kind is a helpful when caring for babies and young children. |

Feeding

Parents will have discussed and decided on either breast- or formula feeding.

Breastfeeding is ideal for a baby and the baby will benefit even if it is only for a few weeks. Help and advice on breastfeeding is available from health visitors and midwives, as well as special breastfeeding counsellors from two organisations, the La Leche League and the National Childbirth Trust. Mothers often find that their own mother, or other mothers who have breastfed their babies, can help them to overcome any problems.

Formula feeding is fine, but parents must ensure that correct amounts are given and strict safety and hygiene precautions are observed during the preparation and storage of feeds.

SAFETY CHECKS

- Check the feed temperature.
- Check that the flow of milk is not too rapid.
- Never force the baby to feed.
- Throw away unused milk.

Things to do

1 Make a list of all the benefits of breastfeeding to a mother and a baby. Can you think of any possible problems?

2 Write down the safety precautions to be taken when preparing and giving formula feeds to a baby.

3 Discuss breastfeeding with a mother who has breastfed her baby. How does she feel about it?

4 Visit local supermarkets or a chemist and make a note of the different types of formula milk and the prices.

_____

_____

_____

_____

_____

_____

_____

_____

_____

_____

_____

_____

_____

_____

Bathing and changing babies

Midwives hold special classes on how to do this at the antenatal clinic. The midwife will also show mothers after the birth. The key things to remember are:

- Prepare everything before fetching and undressing the baby.
- Always check the water temperature.
- Never leave the baby unattended in the bath.

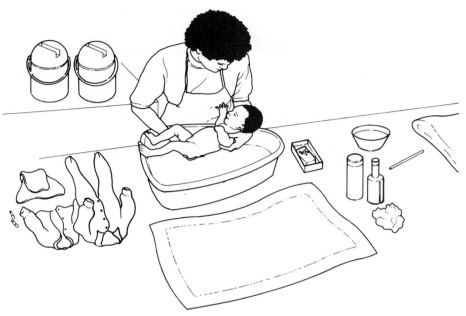

All care procedures are very well described in The Health Education Authority books *Pregnancy* and *Birth to Five*.

Things to do	1	Make a list of the essential equipment needed for bathing and changing a baby.
	2	Visit two different suppliers and compare the prices of the equipment that you have selected.
	3	Work out the weekly cost of disposable nappies for a baby who weighs 7kg.

Equipment and clothing for babies and children

As you can see by looking round supermarkets and specialist children's shops, a huge array of equipment and clothing is available. Parents have plenty of choice, and it is tempting to buy far too many things. In addition, there are financial considerations. Buying for a baby can seriously stretch a family budget. Of course, family and friends will want to buy things for the baby, but nevertheless parents should plan and buy carefully to avoid unnecessary expense. The minimum requirements are shown below.

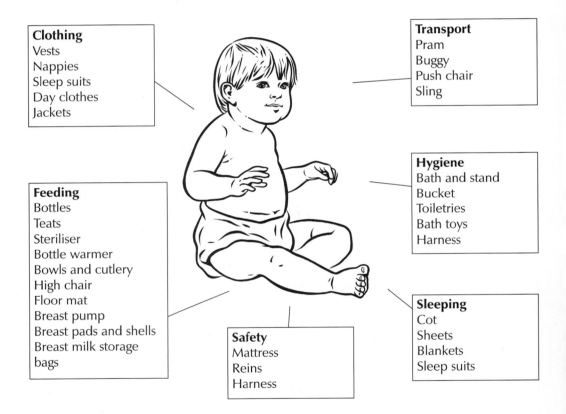

Clothing
Vests
Nappies
Sleep suits
Day clothes
Jackets

Transport
Pram
Buggy
Push chair
Sling

Feeding
Bottles
Teats
Steriliser
Bottle warmer
Bowls and cutlery
High chair
Floor mat
Breast pump
Breast pads and shells
Breast milk storage bags

Hygiene
Bath and stand
Bucket
Toiletries
Bath toys
Harness

Safety
Mattress
Reins
Harness

Sleeping
Cot
Sheets
Blankets
Sleep suits

Essential equipment and clothing for use in baby care

Many people like to use second-hand equipment that has been given by friends and family, or there are very good specialist second-hand shops for baby goods. Always check second-hand equipment carefully before use. As children grow older, the need for physical care equipment becomes less, and parents will find that the need will be to provide toys and stimulating activities.

Things to do

1   Collect as many catalogues of baby equipment as you can, and visit local suppliers.

2   Make a list of points to consider, e.g. cost when choosing equipment for babies.

ASPECTS OF PARENTHOOD

Toys and play

Parents will want to provide toys for their babies and older children.

Play is the way children learn – the more they play, the more they will learn.

However, it's worth remembering that not all play is about playing with toys; children learn from their parents, families and everything that is going on around them, so they need to be talked to and shown interesting things. Children of all ages get bored when they are not learning things.

There are various ways in which parents can help their children learn:

- Have a sense of fun and interest themselves.
- Make the home interesting for babies and children by having mobiles, pictures, day-and-time charts, weather charts and displays of things children have made.
- Include babies and children in day-to-day tasks.

- Communicate right from the start. Babies and older children need to see and talk to parents.
- Enjoy tapes of nursery rhymes and videos of stories with children.
- Give time and attention to what a child wants to do.
- Plan and arrange outings and visits such as shopping, a bus or tram ride, the park, an adventure playground, a farm, swimming.
- Make the home safe and child friendly by moving breakable things out of the way and protecting younger children by using safety gates, drawer and cupboard safety catches, etc.

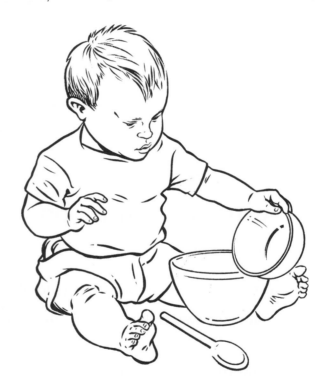

Some household items can make good play equipment

Check out toy safety

- Look for the British Standard kitemark or the CE mark.
- Second-hand toys or toys from car-boot sales can be dangerous.
- Beware of small parts and sharp edges.
- Buy toys that are suitable for the age of the child.

Things to do Make lists of suitable items and toys to interest children of the following ages:

- newborn
- three months
- eight months
- one year
- 18 months
- three years
- five years
- nine years

_____

_____

_____

_____

_____

_____

_____

_____

_____

_____

_____

Measuring progress

During the first year of life, babies develop physically, intellectually, emotionally and socially. At the end of the first year, they will usually have been weaned onto solid foods, be starting to drink from a baby cup and will try to feed themselves. They may have crawled at about nine months of age and walked by their first birthday. They will have started to babble and then say a few words.

Parents may have been keeping a record of this in a special book. Babies will also have regular health and developmental checks at the local clinic or GP surgery. Parents will be asked to keep records of development, medical checks and immunisations given. Records are also kept at the clinic or surgery.

Things to do	1	Did your parents keep a record of your growth and development and the immunisations you were given? See if you can have a look at it.
	2	Do you think recording this kind of information is useful? If so, why?
	3	Find out about the usual programme of immunisations for babies and children and try to obtain a copy of a leaflet giving information.
	4	Find out where can parents get information if they are worried about their child's development or the immunisation programme.

Keeping babies and children safe

Parents and other adults are responsible for keeping babies and children safe. Research has shown that accidents are more likely to occur at certain times and that children are particularly vulnerable. (You will find some information on this in Chapter 1.) Particular dangers in babies can be cot death and choking. Older children will need to be made aware of stranger and road danger.

Parents should know how to give first aid – attending a practical first-aid course is a good idea. There is also some information in Chapter 4.

About cot death

This is Sudden Infant Death Syndrome or SIDS. Unfortunately on rare occasions a baby dies during a period of sleep for no obvious reason. Doctors are not entirely sure why this happens but they do know that certain things seem to reduce the risk of SIDS.

To reduce the risk of cot death

- Baby should sleep on his or her back in the pram, cot or buggy.
- The feet of the baby should touch the bottom end of the cot.
- Sheets and blankets should be positioned so that they cannot be pulled over the baby's face. Duvets and pillows must not be used.

- A room temperature of 18–21° Celsius, depending upon the number of blankets used.
- No smoking anywhere near the baby.
- If the baby is unwell in any way, seek medical advice; it is better to be safe than sorry.

Things to do Make a chart that shows the risks and how they might be prevented for babies and children of the following age groups:

- up to 12 months
- one to three years
- three to five years
- five to ten years
- ten to 16 years.

Possible problems in childhood

There can be problems at each age and stage of development. Some can be serious and may require specialist help. However, sometimes having a bit of knowledge and experience and using common sense is all that is necessary.

Problems in the first year of life include the baby crying, colic, not sleeping, refusing feeds. Toddlers can have eating problems, problems with toilet training, not settling to sleep, not wanting to be left alone. From the age of 18 months temper tantrums may start. Children may kick and bite; some children are overactive; others may be shy and withdrawn. Older children can become nervous and moody.

Things to do 1 Make a list of possible problems at the various stages of development.

2 Discuss possible solutions within your class/group. Note how many times you agree or disagree on a solution.

_____
_____
_____
_____
_____
_____
_____

Discipline

Children need to know that parents love them unconditionally. Parents should give praise and encouragement whenever possible. However, parents and carers must discuss and decide upon ways of dealing with various situations requiring discipline and back each other up when they arise. Of course, everyone has their own ideas about the best ways of handling a temper tantrum: whether they should ignore it, try to distract the child or shout at the child, etc.

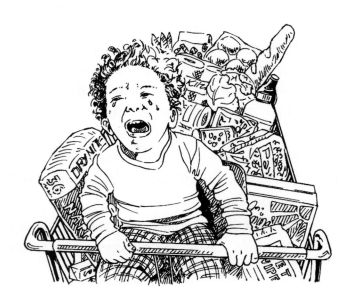

How would you deal with a temper tantrum?

If a parent or carer has definitely said 'no', they should try to stick to what has been said. They should always try to be fair and consistent.

Rewards are not always a good idea. It is best not to promise rewards beforehand. Give one after something has been achieved and remember that a hug counts as a reward.

Smacking children is not helpful, even if it stops them from doing whatever they are doing at that moment. Children learn most by example, so if they are smacked, they think it is acceptable to smack others. Children who are treated aggressively by their parents are more likely to be aggressive themselves.

No one can be a perfect parent, and every parent or carer has bad days. Similarly, children can go through awkward patches, like refusing to dress, eat or go to bed. Sometimes things can be very difficult and may overwhelm parents. This is the time to talk to family and friends and to seek advice from professionals. Parents can talk in confidence about their feelings and problems to organisations such as Parentline, the NSPCC and Parents Anonymous.

Things to do	1	Discuss rewards and punishments within your group/class.
	2	Have a debate on the issue 'Are there any circumstances in which smacking a child is justified?' Vote on the issue within your class/group.

Nobody's perfect

Being a parent is a tremendous privilege. To be responsible for the care of another human being is awesome. It is hard, demanding work, carrying a great responsibility. Some mothers say it is easier to be in full-time employment than to be at home looking after children.

Small children and older children make demands upon parents in different ways. A parent is always a parent, and it doesn't end when the child is 17.

At the end of the day, neither parents nor children are perfect. As parents gain experience, they become more confident and become even better parents. Children who grow up in a loving secure environment where there are opportunities to learn and develop are well equipped to face adult life.

6 The Family

WHAT IS THE FAMILY?

Most people understand that the word *family* refers to those who may be related to each other by blood or adoption, by marriage or arrangement. There is a general notion that a family consists of mother, father, brothers and sisters, but there are many variations on this pattern.

There are many ways in which the family can be organised and still carry out the basic tasks. In Britain monogamy (one man–one wife) is the only legal form of marriage, but in some countries one woman may have several husbands (polyandry) or one man may have several wives (polygamy).

In Israel, there is a very different type of support network, called the *kibbutz*. Here, children live in special children's houses looked after by a mother substitute and only spend a limited time with their parents. Men and women, freed from childcare responsibilities, work on farms and in factories.

In Britain, it is often possible to identify members of an 'immediate' or 'nuclear' family in the centre of a wider family setting. The members of the wider, or 'extended', family may be aunts, uncles, cousins or grandparents. Members of the extended family may live some distance from the nuclear family, and this may make frequent contact more difficult, but relationships may still be close. People may keep in touch via phone, e-mail and visits.

Things to do	1	Think about a family you know (it may be a single-carer family, a family with step-sisters or -brothers or a step-parent). Write down who you think belongs to it. Compare what you have written with other group members.
	2	Think about a family you know and write down the members of the *immediate* family and the members of the *extended* family.

_____

_____

_____

_____

_____

_____

_____

_____

_____

_____

WHAT DO FAMILIES DO?

New members of society need to be socialised into the patterns of behaviour, values and rules of that society. Professionals could do this (and sometimes families need professional support: see *Services to support families* on page 111), but throughout history, the family has had the responsibility of passing on the culture of the society to the children. The form of the family may have changed considerably, but the tasks and the functions of the family still continue. Families still bring up children as they have done for centuries. This process is called *socialisation* and it is something that each individual goes through. Children learn how to be part of society in the first place through those that care for them. Families help them to talk, they guide their behaviour and children often become what is expected of them. Of course, sometimes they don't and this can lead to tension between parents and children.

Socialisation doesn't stop with childhood and doesn't just involve parents/carers. Socialisation goes on throughout life, influenced by friends, school, media and work.

Another of the family's tasks is reproduction. The family structure is one way of bringing children into the world and providing them with what they need to grow physically, emotionally and socially.

Possible advantages of living in a family

If a young child doesn't have a 'family' upbringing, like a young girl called Genie, who was locked in a room to fend for herself with only food and a bucket to use as a toilet, they will have problems fitting in to society. Genie's was an extreme case, but most people can appreciate the value of family life both in a practical sense and because of how we feel when we are separated from our families or when a family member is ill or in trouble.

Possible disadvantages of family life

If the family works well, it can be a tremendous source of support and a very positive force in developing children's personalities; but we all know that families aren't positive all of the time. Some carers may be abusive and damaging to their children. They may neglect them. Some children can be hard on their parents and hard with each other. Settled families may break up. There may be denial of opportunities, pressure on children to succeed or earn money. Some parents may be 'too soft' or indulgent with their children. Sometimes, pressures outside the family, like low income, unemployment, poor health, bereavement (deep sadness when someone dies), accidents or stress at work, cause family tensions which may be very difficult to overcome.

Things to do	1	Think about a family you know. What do they do for each other?
	2	Think about your own background. Can you remember some of the things your parents/carers said to you? Discuss your memories in small groups and reflect on what your parents/carers said and how that may have affected you.

'Be careful when you cross the road.'
'Yes, mother, I will, I'm 27 now! I'll manage.'

Practical advantages of family life

- Provides:
  - basic needs, such as food and shelter
  - care when ill
  - protection
  - a place to rest, relax and play
- Enables tasks to be shared (division of labour)

Social and emotional advantages of family life

- Provides:
  - support
  - company
  - socialisation (see opposite)
  - education
  - stimulation
  - a place to escape and be yourself
  - love, security and attention
  - an introduction to wider relationships
  - fairness and discipline
- Prepares children for school and work
- Teaches children to care, share, give and receive

Practical disadvantages of family life

- Insufficient provision for basic needs
- Some members of the family are overburdened (unfair division of labour)
- Poor housing
- Too little income

Social disadvantages of family life

- Narrow range of experience
- Opportunities for improvement denied
- Inconsistency of discipline: strict/indulgent
- Dominant adults impose too much on children
- Tense atmosphere
- Anxiety
- Anger
- Violence

Emotional disadvantages of family life

- No fun
- No stimulation
- Children have low self-esteem

Things to do

1 Look at the list below. Think about a family you know and make a note of who does each job. In some families, the work tasks are very separate and members are very clear about what they are expected to do. In other families, there may be less clarity. How does it work in the family you know?

- decorates the house
- provides income
- cleans the house
- shops for food
- pays the bills
- does the gardening
- mends a washer or a fuse
- washing
- reminds family members to write thank you letters/be polite
- cleans the car
- takes the car for its MOT
- arranges family outings or people to visit
- arranges holidays
- helps with homework
- looks after young children
- looks after older relatives
- looks after family members when they are ill
- organises family events (like weddings or parties)
- talks with family members when they are upset or disappointed

2 Now think about the following:

- How interconnected are these roles? For example, if one carer doesn't earn a wage, does the other carer have greater difficulty organising a family holiday?
- What role do other services outside the family play?
- What difference does the number of children make to the workload in a family? (Do older children help in your family?)

- What support do you give and gain practically and emotionally in your family?
- What difference do you think the age of the children makes to the amount and types of workload within the family?
- What kind of support can older members give the family?

_____

_____

_____

_____

_____

_____

Older members of the family can be very supportive when children are very young; yet these older members may need support themselves with increasing age.

'My gran always comes every Saturday night. She used to come to babysit for us when we were young. Now that we're older, we're all off out, but she still likes to come for her tea and the change. She used to make our tea, now we make hers. In fact, she's very fond of Chinese takeaways.'

Family change

Life doesn't allow for action replays. You can't go back, you have to continue in the process of change and development. Change may seem more important at particular points in our lives, like starting school, leaving school to go to work, getting married, having a baby. These major change points are sometimes called transitions. Obviously as family members go through periods of *transition*, relationships within the family setting will be affected and sometimes tested.

FAMILY RELATIONSHIPS

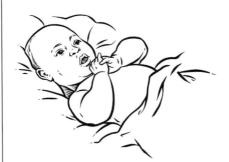

- New parents have to adjust to possible sleepless nights

- There is extra work considering the baby's needs before their own needs.

- Older family members may help.

- New parents gain joy, hope, pride and purpose.

- Adolescents may feel the pressure of seeking out further education, work and new relationships.

- There is the interest and excitement of new possibilities and growing independence.

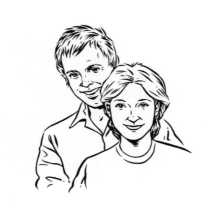

- Young adults may be leaving home, finding partners; sadness at family members leaving, but joy with the addition of family members' partners.

- Time for parental couple to spend together.

- Time to take up new hobbies and interests or revive old ones.

- Growing dependence and/or increasing need of older relatives.

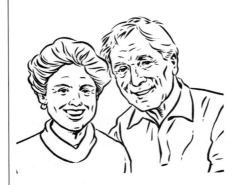

- Opportunity to repay earlier work and support given.

- Opportunity for respect, thankful for the lives and wisdom of these older people.

- Older people may have time to talk and reflect with other members or listen to them.

Just as people are continually changing, being socialised by and for new and different situations, so it is inevitable that the relationships they form need to change. Transition times often test relationships.

Relationships change not only because individuals change and develop, but also because of wider issues – a woman may return to work because her husband loses his job, a family member may become ill or someone may change jobs and move to a different part of the country.

Things to do

1 Look at the comments below and think about what type of change or transition might have provoked them.

'I thought Charlie was such a darling until he reached the age of two.'

'I can't do a thing right since she's started school. Even the location of the spaghetti on the plate seems wrong.'

'I have to walk behind her now that she is in the Juniors. She doesn't like the idea of me taking her to school.'

'He wants to choose his own clothes now he is in secondary school.'

'Every time she goes in that bathroom, she slams the door and locks it. She is ages in there fiddling about with her hair – at 14! I ask you!

'She doesn't know what to do with herself. She wants to go to college, but she isn't that confident. She sounds off a lot at home, but that's just at me and her dad. We don't matter.'

'I used to enjoy going to see my dad, but he has become so confused lately.'

2 Think about the transition points of the members of the family that you know. In what ways may family relationships be under attack?

3 Think about each family member:
- Do they help practically with tasks around the house or by earning to support the family?
- Do they help emotionally by considering another person?
- Do they help socially by keeping the peace, organising treats, contributing to family occasions?

Family culture

Every family is unique. Every family has different ways of living out their life together. And no family stays the same, because no child or person stays the same.

Things to do	In small groups, discuss the following statements in relation to a family you know and compare your findings. Keep a note for your assessment evidence.
	The family I know is …
	    • small and closely knit – there are only (four) members;
	    • large with many children; gran and granddad live with the main family;
	    • large because it includes several step-children;
	    • interesting because the parents are also foster parents;
	    • hectic – the parents are registered childminders;
	    • a single-carer family.
	The family I know has …
	    • arguments;
	    • fun times;
	    • good holidays;
	    • celebrations;
	    • meals out;
	    • Eid together;
	    • Christmas together;
	    • Sunday dinner together.
	In the family I know, …
	    • the men do the cooking;
	    • the women take care of the children;
	    • the household tasks are shared;
	    • everyone says their prayers;
	    • the men go to the mosque on a Friday evening;
	    • everyone goes to church.

FAMILY FESTIVALS AND SPECIAL FOOD

Most people enjoy food and company. There may have been a mealtime you enjoyed very much – perhaps eating out with friends. It may be helpful to try to work out why you remember it and why it was special for you. Often family gatherings involve eating together.

Things to do	Make a list of the times when a family you know comes together. Who usually prepares the food? Is there a special meal? Is there a traditional pattern of events surrounding the meal? For example, at Eid, do people visit other family members before eating? At Christmas, does the family go to church?

Food rules

Many religions have rules that govern what their followers may eat. There are also foods that are traditionally eaten at festival times. The following sections provide information about some of these rules and the foods associated with different religious festivals.

Jewish custom

In strict Jewish households, people prepare and eat only *kosher* food. *Kosher* means 'right or fit to eat'. Kosher meat does not contain blood. The meat is drained of blood by a particular method of slaughtering and a process of salting. The opposite of kosher is *trefah*, which means forbidden. Certain meat, fish and poultry are trefah. Another law forbids the mixing of meat and milk in both the preparation and the ingredients. In Jewish households where this law is observed, separate utensils and crockery may be used for the two elements.

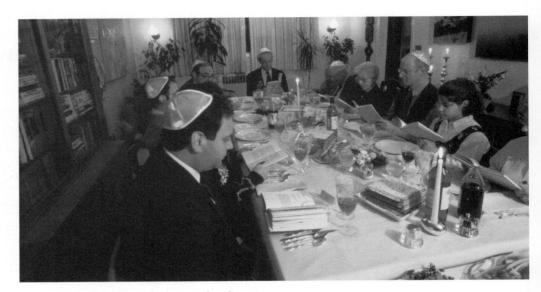

A Jewish family praying before Seder dinner

Things to do	1	Find out about the following breads:

- matzo;
- Sabbath;
- latke;
- challah.

2 Find out what the following Jewish festivals celebrate:

- Seder;
- Hanukkah;
- Rosh Hashanah;
- Yom Kippur.

Islamic custom

Like Jews, Muslims do not eat pork and only eat meat that has been slaughtered and prepared in a certain way, in Arabic *halal*. Food that is not permitted is called *haram*. Halal foods do not contain any pig products. This includes cakes and sweets if they contain animal fat.

The need for these food laws often have practical reasons behind them. The belief of some religions that certain foods are 'unclean' and can be harmful may originate from the climate or conditions prevailing at the time the rules were laid down. Sometimes the food laws are to remind people of God and sometimes they are to prevent people from eating with unbelievers.

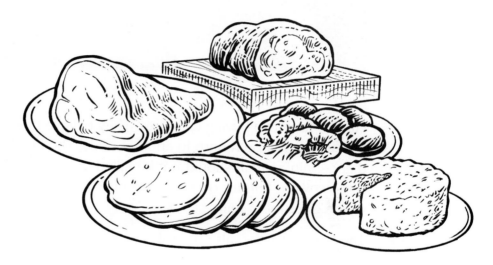

Ham, bacon and shellfish are some of the foods forbidden in Islamic custom

Muslims fast during the month of Ramadan, when nothing is eaten from sunrise to sunset. After sunset, many Muslims follow the example of the prophet Muhammad and eat a date with a drink of water. Children are not expected to fast, but often go without sweets and snacks as training for the adult fast. The fasting reminds the Muslim people of their faith and also brings the community together because everyone fasts, whether they are rich or poor. At the end of Ramadan, there is great celebration at the festival of Eid-ul-Fitr. The celebration lasts for three days. People visit their relatives and friends and eat the special foods that have been prepared. Children enjoy traditional sweets and gifts of money from relatives.

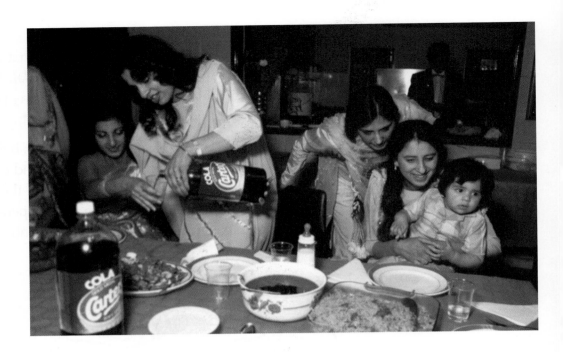

Hindu custom

Hindus respect all living creatures. They believe that all living things have a soul which will be reborn in another body. The Hindu tradition teaches that certain animals should not be killed and eaten. One of these animals is the cow, so Hindus do not eat beef. They see no reason to eat an animal which gives them milk.

The Hindu religion also has rules which specify who may prepare food for others. This may be based on the idea of castes. Although most Hindu people do not live within the caste system any more, the system strictly separates groups of people and determines the sort of job a person may do or whom they are able to marry. A low-caste person would only be able to do quite menial or low-skilled work and could only marry someone of the same caste.

Many religions recognise the importance of food, and it may play an important part in religious services. During a Hindu service, the priest may place milk and sweets on a tray with purified water, incense and a lamp. The food is offered to the gods and then shared out among the worshippers. The food becomes holy food when it is shared and is called *prashad*. As part of the service, water and milk are placed in the worshipper's right hand with a spoon. After a special weekly service called *Havan*, the worshippers join together for a vegetarian meal. At Diwali, the birthdays of many gods are remembered, and people eat sweet foods to celebrate. Often molasses (a rich, dark-brown, treacly substance which can be used to enrich bread made with dark flour) is used in recipes because the gods Rama and Krishna enjoyed this food.

Many Hindu people sprinkle water over their food and ask God to bless it. A small amount of the food may be taken for animals or birds. Hindus take great care to keep food away from dirt, and any leftover food is thrown away. Many people wash their hands after eating, but for Muslims, Hindus and Sikhs, this can have religious importance as well.

Things to do	Find some recipes that include molasses as an ingredient.

Sikh custom

Strict Sikhs may say a prayer whilst preparing food. Women cover their heads whilst preparing or serving food, and some may take a bath to make sure they are clean before food preparation. There should be no gossip in the Sikh temple, the *gurdwara*, whilst food is being prepared.

Like Jews and Muslims, Sikhs have their own way of killing animals for food. Followers of the Sikh religion do not eat beef, even though the teachings of their gurus do not forbid it. Many Sikhs say prayers before food. In the gurdwara, Sikhs cover their heads as a sign of respect, hold a *chapati* in their hands and say prayers.

Sikhs share a food called *karah parshad*, which is a mixture of butter, sugar and water prepared in a ritual way. A prayer is said and a special sword is used to mix the ingredients. The Sikh teacher Guru Nanak invited people to eat in the temple together to show that everyone is equal. This act also symbolises how strong a community that eats and worships together can be.

Christian custom

The main way in which food is involved in the Christian religion is through the celebration of the Lord's Supper or Holy Communion. During this service, Christians prepare themselves with prayers and readings and say sorry to God for their sins (the *confession*), and the priest, vicar or minister blesses some bread and wine (Baptist and Methodist churches have non-alcoholic wine). The congregation gathers around a focal point (usually a table), or in some churches the wine and bread are brought to the people by the minister and some assistants. They eat a small piece of the bread and drink a small amount of the wine to remember the body and blood of Jesus Christ who died so that people could have peace with God. The bread and wine symbolise the body and blood of Christ.

Some Christian people fast on *Ash Wednesday*, the beginning of Lent. Lent is the period of 40 days which commemorates the time Jesus spent fasting in the wilderness. Some people give up certain foods during this time as a discipline and preparation for Easter.

Some Christians eat only fish on *Good Friday*, the day of Christ's crucifixion, as the fish was the secret symbol of the Christian faith. At Easter, Christians remember the resurrection of Jesus, and rich foods, simnel cakes and chocolate eggs are eaten. The eggs also represent new life.

Similarly at *Christmas*, the birth of Jesus is celebrated. Christians have a special holiday and often eat a traditional meal of turkey and rich fruit pudding.

There are many different food rituals, just as there are many forms of the family. It is also true that within the Jewish culture, for example, there are many degrees of Jewishness; some believers may be strict, others less so. This could also be said of Muslims, Hindus, Sikhs and Christians. Perhaps the one common theme is that people do come together to eat, even if only on special occasions, or with only the company of the television.

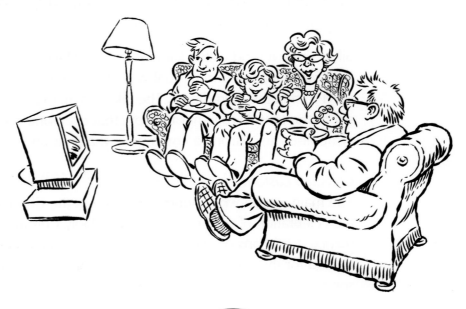

Things to do	In small groups, prepare a wall chart to show the foods that are used in services in synagogues, mosques, temples and churches. Use books from the library and visit websites to obtain information. Discuss together what these foods symbolise.

SERVICES TO SUPPORT FAMILIES

The 1989 Children Act

The 1989 Children Act recognized that children need their families, and local authorities have a duty to help families bring up children who could be called 'in need'. Children in need may have learning difficulties, a physical disability or a poor home life.

Social workers are involved with families when children are assessed as being 'in need'. They may also be involved if there is any concern that children may be 'at risk' from harm or neglect.

The Act states that children under five in need are entitled to daycare. This may be in the form of a nursery place.

The Act stated that local authorities must inspect any arrangements or establishment where children are looked after for more than two hours. This includes:

- playgroups;
- childminders;
- crèches;
- nurseries;
- children's homes or family group homes;
- schools where children stay (residential schools).

Once a place is inspected and registered, the registration lasts for one year. It is an offence to look after children in settings that are not registered. Since April 2001 the inspection body OFSTED which inspects schools and colleges also inspects pre-school provision. Establishments which fail inspection may not be able to remain open.

Health services

The following services are free for all children up to the age of 16, or 18 if they remain in full-time education:

- prescriptions;
- eye checkups;
- dental checkups.

Pregnant women also receive free prescriptions and dental check-ups throughout the pregnancy and the first year following the birth;

There are *statutory* services (services which people are entitled to by law) provided by the government, through local authorities. Services may also be provided by voluntary or charitable groups. Note that *voluntary* refers to the status of the organisation; it does not mean that all the workers are unpaid. Some services are provided on a commercial basis, meaning that the organisers need to make a profit from the establishment. The various services are outlined below.

Primary Healthcare Team
The team consists of:

- Midwife: works with the GP and gives *antenatal* care (takes care of a woman's health before she has the baby).
- Health visitor: visits mother and baby when the midwife has finished. He/She carries out routine checks on the baby and advises the mother about matters like feeding and weaning. In some areas, health visitors also visit older family members.
- GP: provides medical treatment and advice. The Practice Nurse may see patients for more minor treatments after the doctor's diagnosis or during 'Well Man/Woman' clinics.

Hospitals or Trusts
People often go to hospitals because a GP has referred them or recommended they should have further help or treatment. This is known as secondary care because it follows the primary or first stage.

Other services
- School Health Service: provides routine checks and immunisation.
- Community Services – district nurse, physiotherapist, hospital transport.

Education

The education services available include:

- nurseries;
- playgroups;
- after-school clubs;
- holiday play schemes;
- primary schools for children aged four to 11;
- secondary schools for pupils aged 11 to 16 or 18;
- further education for students aged 16 or over.

Schools are also provided for children who have additional needs. The 1981 Education Act encouraged the integration of children with additional needs into mainstream schools. This is reinforced by the Disability Discrimination Acts, 1995, 2000 and eventually 2004.

Things to do

Choose five items from the list below and find out where these services are in your area. Find out whether the service is statutory, voluntary, commercial or independent. Warning! It isn't always easy to find out the exact body which is responsible for the service, because sometimes both the responsibility and the funding (who pays for the service) is shared, in a partnership arrangement.

You may be able to ask neighbours and friends with children. Others in your group may know, and there are formal organisations, such as libraries and Children's Information Services, which will help.

- Parent and baby group
- Toddler group
- Baby clinic
- Day nursery
- Playgroup
- Nursery
- Infant school
- After school club
- Story-telling sessions

- Music-making groups
- Gym clubs
- Indoor adventure place
- Outdoor recreation place
- Library
- Museum
- Art gallery
- Art/craft classes or workshops
- Uniformed groups (e.g. Rainbows, Cubs and Scouts)
- Swimming pools*
- Evening classes
- Job centre
- Community centre

*If you choose this option, try to find out also special times or sessions for children's lessons or women-only sessions. Some pools set aside particular times for people with disabilities. Obviously people with disabilities should be able to go with everyone else, but some may enjoy a quieter session.

Benefits

Various benefits are available to support families. These include:

- Child Benefit;
- Child Support Agency;
- Single Parent Benefit;
- Education Maintenance Allowance;
- Working Family Tax Credit.

Some benefits are *contributory*. This means they can only be paid if the person has paid enough National Insurance contributions from their income. Contributory benefits include Maternity Pay, Widowed Mother's Allowance and Job Seekers allowance. No contributions are necessary for payment of non-contributory benefits, but the person must be entitled to receive them. Lone Parent Benefit, Child Benefit and Housing Benefit are all *non-contributory* benefits.

Some benefits are *means tested*, which means the person has to state all other income and savings. The benefit is then adjusted accordingly. People may be entitled to benefits but not claim them because either they may not know that they *can* claim or they may feel too proud to claim. Sometimes the claim forms for the benefits are difficult for some people to manage.

Things to do	Collect benefit booklets from the Post Office or Citizen's Advice Bureau and check who can claim these benefits and how much they amount to. See if you can find any information in community languages, i.e. in languages other than English.

Housing

Local authorities have a duty to provide homeless people in their area with accommodation, and families are a priority. Rent officers are employed by local authorities to check whether rents are fair and to help sort out difficulties between people renting (*tenants*) and people owning the property (*landlords*).

Voluntary organisations and children

There are many organisations that aim to support the needs of children and their families. Here are a few of them:
- NSPCC (The National Society for the Prevention of Cruelty to Children)
- PLA (The Pre-School Learning Alliance)
- Barnardos
- The Children's Society
- The Save the Children Fund
- After-School Clubs

Things to do	Find out what these organisations do and if there is a branch near to you.

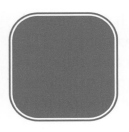

Appendix

Daily care routine for a 3-month-old baby

Time	What happens	Need	Response/Outcome
0600	Baby wakes up crying.	Human contact and affection.	Talk to baby and give a cuddle.
	Nappy is wet and soiled.	To be clean and comfortable.	Remove soiled nappy, clean baby and put on a clean nappy. Talk to baby while this is done.
0615	Baby making sucking sounds and crying loudly.	A breast or bottle feed.	Give breast or bottle feed.
0630	Baby is awake and restless.	Social contact and affection.	Cuddle and talk to, or play with, baby.
0645	Baby looks sleepy.	Sleep.	Put to sleep in cot on back or side, feet at bottom of cot.
0930	Baby wakes and cries. Nappy is wet. Baby is hungry.	To be comforted. To be made clean and comfortable. A breast or bottle feed. Social contact and affection.	Cuddle. Speak to softly. Wash face and hands. Change nappy. Dress in daytime outfit. Give a breast or bottle feed. Play with cot toys, while talking or singing to baby.
1100	Baby rubbing eyes and looking tired.	Sleep.	Place baby safely in cot or pram for a sleep.
1400	Baby awake. Nappy wet and soiled. Hungry.	Contact with carer. Nappy change. Breast or bottle feed. Interaction/play. Fresh air.	Cuddle, talk, smile. Change nappy. Give breast or bottle feed. Place baby in pram ready for walk to park or shops. More baby/carer interaction. Allow baby to sleep in pram.

1700	Baby in pram waking up from a sleep.	To have a drink of diluted juice or water from a bottle. To have a bath. To change into night clothes. To have a breast or bottle feed. To talk and play with carer. To settle in cot for sleep. To be comforted and cuddled. To have a clean nappy.	Talk to baby. Give baby a drink of dilute juice or water. Bath baby, using opportunity for further play and interaction. Feed baby. Talk to baby, cuddle and prepare for bed. Settle baby in cot in recommended position for sleep.
2200	Baby wakes crying, wet nappy and hungry.	To have a breast or bottle feed. To be settled in cot to sleep. To be changed, comforted and fed.	Comfort and cuddle baby. Change nappy. Feed baby. Settle baby in cot for sleep.
0200	Baby wakes.	To be comforted and possibly fed and changed. To be settled in cot to sleep.	Comfort, change, feed if necessary. As babies grow older they may not wake at this time.

Daily care routine for an 85-year-old woman

Time	What happens	Need	Response/Outcome
0600	Joan has been lying awake in bed for 2 hours; she would like to go to the toilet but finds it difficult on her own. Her carer will not arrive until 7 a.m.	To see and hear more clearly. To be helped to walk to the toilet so that she can pass urine.	Joan puts her glasses on and places her hearing aid in her ear without assistance.
0700	Wants to pass urine and have a wash. Would love a cup of tea and a chat to someone.	Assistance required to help her to toilet. Assistance with washing. To put dentures in mouth. Drink of tea. To talk to someone.	Home carer arrives and takes her to the bathroom where she is able to use the toilet and have a good wash. Puts dentures in without help. The carer and Joan have a cup of tea and a chat together.

0720	Joan wants to get dressed and have her breakfast.	Help with dressing. Help with food preparation.	The carer helps Joan to choose the clothes she will wear and assists with dressing. The carer asks Joan what she would like for breakfast and then makes it for her.
0830	The bedclothes need changing. There is a lot of soiled linen and clothing.	Help with household tasks, changing bed and washing clothes.	The carer changes the bed and puts all the dirty washing together so that it can be taken to the launderette to be washed.
0930	Joan sits in a chair by an electric fire; she is cold and bored. She needs something to do until lunchtime.	Warmth. Comfort. Something to do. Something to eat and drink.	Carer gives Joan a rug for her knees. Daily paper is delivered for Joan to read. Carer sets up anglepoise lamp so that Joan can see to read and do the crossword more easily. Carer leaves a flask of coffee and a biscuit for mid-morning snack.
1045	Neighbour arrives, offers to do shopping and collect pension.	Company. Shopping. Pension collection.	Neighbour has a chat about local events. Neighbour collects pension and shopping.
1115	Joan is uncomfortable sitting. Wants to pass urine. Joan is hungry.	To move about to ease aching joints. To use the toilet. A hot meal.	No care given. Joan manages on her own using a room frame to help her to walk. Carer then arrives and heats up a pre-prepared meal in the microwave, serves the food, then clears away.
1230	Joan wants to go to the toilet.	To move about. To go to the toilet.	Carer helps Joan to toilet and assists with washing hands.

1300	Joan would like a nap by the fire.	Sleep in warmth and comfort.	Carer settles Joan in chair by fire, covers knees with a rug. Carer leaves everything to hand including a flask of tea and a piece of cake.
1500	Joan wakes up. Wants a drink and a snack. Wants something to do. Wants to use the toilet.	Drink. Snack. Something to do. To go to the toilet.	Drinks the tea and eats the cake left by the carer. Watches daytime TV; the carer has left the remote control within reach. Manages to get to toilet and wash hands using the room frame for support.
1600	Wants something to do. Wants some company.	Something to do to relieve boredom. A visitor.	Finishes crossword puzzle she started earlier. Joan's daughter calls on the way home from work and they have a chat about what she has been doing.
1800	Hungry. Wants to go to the toilet.	Evening meal. To pass urine.	Carer arrives and heats up a pre-prepared meal in the microwave, serves the food, then clears away and leaves. Joan manages to get to toilet and wash her hands using the room frame for support.
1845	Bored.	To be entertained.	Sits in chair by fire and watches TV, Channel 4 news, then soaps (*Coronation Street* and *Brookside*).
1900	Thirsty.	To have a drink.	Drinks a milk stout* which the carer has left ready.

* Milk stout: a stout (beer) drink made with lactose

Time	Activity	Need	Carer action
2000	Wants to use the toilet.	To pass urine. To be washed.	Carer assists with this and helps Joan to bed leaving a commode nearby.
2100	Wants to go to sleep.	To be settled for sleep.	Carer leaves a drink of water. Leaves radio within reach. Carer checks that alarm button is functioning, says good night and leaves, locking the door.
2130		Remove teeth, glasses and hearing aid.	Removes teeth, glasses and hearing aid by herself.
2300	Goes to sleep after listening to the radio.		

Index